Fueling Young Athletes

Heather R. Mangieri, RDN, CSSD, MS

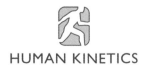

HUMAN KINETICS

Library of Congress Cataloging-in-Publication Data

Names: Mangieri, Heather R., 1974- author.
Title: Fueling young athletes / Heather R. Mangieri.
Description: Champaign, IL : Human Kinetics, [2017] | Includes
bibliographical references and index.
Identifiers: LCCN 2016025735 (print) | LCCN 2016038883 (ebook) | ISBN
9781492522096 (print) | ISBN 9781492531449 (ebook)
Subjects: LCSH: Nutrition--Popular works. | Athletes--Nutrition--Popular
works. | Exercise--Physiological aspects--Popular works.
Classification: LCC RA784 .M2956 2017 (print) | LCC RA784 (ebook) | DDC
613.2088/796--dc23
LC record available at https://lccn.loc.gov/2016025735

ISBN: 978-1-4925-2209-6 (print)

This publication is written and published to provide accurate and authoritative information relevant to the subject matter presented. It is published and sold with the understanding that the author and publisher are not engaged in rendering legal, medical, or other professional services by reason of their authorship or publication of this work. If medical or other expert assistance is required, the services of a competent professional person should be sought.

Notice: Permission to reproduce the following material is granted to instructors and agencies who have purchased *Fueling Young Athletes:* pp. 59, 60, 141, 143-145, 152. The reproduction of other parts of this book is expressly forbidden by the above copyright notice. Persons or agencies who have not purchased *Fueling Young Athletes* may not reproduce any material.

The web addresses cited in this text were current as of August 2016, unless otherwise noted.

Acquisitions Editor: Michelle Maloney; **Developmental Editor:** Laura Pulliam; **Managing Editor:** Nicole Moore; **Copyeditor:** Patsy Fortney; **Proofreader:** Jan Feeney; **Indexer:** Dan Connolly; **Permissions Manager:** Martha Gullo; **Graphic Designer:** Tara Welsch and Angela K. Snyder; **Cover Designer:** Keith Blomberg; **Photograph (cover):** Jason Allen; **Photo Asset Manager:** Laura Fitch; **Photo Production Manager:** Jason Allen; **Senior Art Manager:** Kelly Hendren; **Illustrations:** © Human Kinetics; **Printer:** Versa Press

Nutritional analyses in chapters 10 and 11 from The Food Processor® Nutrition and Fitness Software 11.2, © 2016 ESHA Research, Inc.

Printed in the United States of America   10   9   8   7   6   5   4   3   2   1

The paper in this book is certified under a sustainable forestry program.

Human Kinetics

Website: www.HumanKinetics.com

United States: Human Kinetics
P.O. Box 5076
Champaign, IL 61825-5076
800-747-4457
e-mail: info@hkusa.com

Canada: Human Kinetics
475 Devonshire Road Unit 100
Windsor, ON N8Y 2L5
800-465-7301 (in Canada only)
e-mail: info@hkcanada.com

Europe: Human Kinetics
107 Bradford Road
Stanningley
Leeds LS28 6AT, United Kingdom
+44 (0) 113 255 5665
e-mail: hk@hkeurope.com

Australia: Human Kinetics
57A Price Avenue
Lower Mitcham, South Australia 5062
08 8372 0999
e-mail: info@hkaustralia.com

New Zealand: Human Kinetics
P.O. Box 80
Mitcham Shopping Centre, South Australia 5062
0800 222 062
e-mail: info@hknewzealand.com

E6706

To my three monsters, Matt, Luke, and Mia, for keeping me grounded in what really matters in life. You three are my everything, and I love you more than words can say.

Contents

Preface

I remember the first athlete I worked with after earning a master's degree in wellness and human performance from the University of Pittsburgh. I was already a registered dietitian with years of experience working with active people, but I now understood the complexity of exercise physiology and sport nutrition on a deeper level. A colleague at the university at which I taught referred this athlete to me; her mom was concerned about her nutrition. Tammy was a 14-year-old competitive soccer player who was nursing her second fracture. Her parents were very supportive of her activities and believed they were doing all the right things to keep her well nourished.

As I reviewed her food journal, I immediately noticed nutritional shortfalls: She was not consuming enough calcium, vitamin D, iron, and many other key nutrients needed to keep her active body strong. I visualized her bones being stripped of calcium and her red blood cells not holding enough of the protein hemoglobin. She needed a diet makeover, and a registered dietitian specializing in sport nutrition was the person to help her. We worked together on a plan that first provided the nutrition she needed for proper growth and development, and then we added the nutrients she needed to improve her sport performance. With time and the right nutrition, Tammy healed, remained injury free, and improved her performance.

Being a good athlete requires more than just eating the right foods before, during, and after an event. Proper diet plays a critical role in keeping athletes free of illness and injury so they can train properly. Training can cause inflammation and pain; the right diet, however, can help build a strong immune system and skeleton and keep you feeling energized, resulting in high-quality training and performance.

Once day-to-day dietary needs are met, it's time to optimize the training diet. The nutrition plan supports the training plan. When athletes eat the right foods in the right amounts at the right times, they can train hard and are in a good position to reach their goals.

When I started my private practice as a sport dietitian, I had no idea I would become so focused on high school athletes. I assumed I would be helping mostly collegiate athletes because that was the group I had the most experience with in training. I do work with college athletes (e.g., baseball players who want to lose weight so they can run faster, hockey players who need help understanding what to eat and drink to prevent fatigue), but it was my work with younger athletes that I found most rewarding. I could relate to their questions and needs from my own experiences. I could help not only because I'm a registered dietitian who is board certified in sport dietetics and understand the science of nutrition, but also because I'm a mother of three, including a swimmer and a competitive cheerleader. I understand the demands of a busy family, the needs of competitive athletes, and the science of how nutrients work to keep us healthy and strong. I relate to the hectic lifestyles of busy parents trying to figure out how to feed a family when each member is running in a different direction. I prepare meals, plan meals in advance, and eat on the go. Packing a cooler with food for the day is my reality. I have a freezer full of ice packs in every shape and size imaginable. But I more than just live it; I have it figured out. I can help, and I love doing it. Working with younger athletes, the ones who need to learn about nutrition not only for proper growth and development, but also to perform better in their sports, is my passion.

The number of children participating in high school sports has increased significantly over the past 20 years. Even more significant is the age at which these children begin sports. I now see athletes as young as eight years old whose parents hire me to help them learn how to fuel their kids. This presents an early opportunity to teach families proper nutrition for health, development, and sport performance.

Teaching athletes at a younger age prepares them to enter adulthood with sound nutrition skills. As such, they are already ahead of the game and have a winning advantage. They are healthy and recognize that food helps them feel good and perform well not just in sports but also in school. Whether these young athletes go on to be collegiate or professional athletes is unknown, but either way, I teach them life skills that help them to be healthy adults. That is one of the most rewarding parts of my career.

As a sport dietitian, I am hired for a variety of reasons. Some young athletes want to change their body composition (lose weight or gain lean muscle mass). Some are having nutrition issues, such as fatigue during practice or bone fractures that won't heal. Parents seek my advice and services because their young athletes have decided to become vegetarian or remove substances such as gluten from their diets. And many of my athletes have disordered eating or are struggling with understanding mixed messages from the media. My goal as a national media spokesperson and an expert in sport nutrition is to break down the science of nutrition into meaningful messages that athletes, parents, and coaches can understand.

This book offers simple and straightforward answers to the questions of why, what, when, where, and how much to eat and drink. It reviews nutrition basics as well as the current scientific evidence on the best sport nutrition practices while answering many of the recurring questions I receive from athletes, parents, and coaches. It also helps athletes understand why adequate sleep is critical to recovery and should be a top priority. This book is the next best thing to a one-on-one consultation to develop an individualized training plan.

Acknowledgments

It is hard to express in words how grateful I am to all of those who inspired, guided, and supported me during the process of writing this book.

A huge thank-you to my amazing kids: Luke, Matthew, and Mia. Without the three of you, my life would be downright boring. Together, we get it done and I love every single moment of it. You three are my entire world. I love you each so much.

To my parents, Tom and Linda Wilson, who set me up for success from a very young age and never stopped supporting or believing in me.

To my brother, Eric Wilson, who triggered the author in me when he spoke the words "You should write a book" when I was just 24 years old. I might have blown you off at that time, but that moment stuck and your words never left my mind. Thank you for boosting my confidence during the early years.

To my best friend, Michelle Lewis, for your unconditional love, friendship, and support in every aspect of my life. You truly are the wind beneath my wings. I love you.

To all of my new and old friends, colleagues, interns, and fellow sport dietitians who have contributed quotations and feedback, given encouragement, tested my recipes, and made sure to keep me active during the writing process. I am grateful for your friendship and support in helping me bring this book to life. A special thanks to Manuel Villacorta, RD. I am grateful for your friendship and guidance and forever blessed that our paths crossed. To Marjorie Nolan Cohn, Linda Samuels, Todd Murray, and Jeremy Hoy, who took extra time to read, edit, organize, and provide valuable insight, feedback, and support from the very beginning of this project. You each hold a unique and special place in my heart and I am forever grateful.

To all of the athletes and their families who have allowed me into their lives and shared their challenges and successes with me. This book truly is for you.

A huge thank you to my entire team at Human Kinetics, especially my team of editors, Michelle Maloney, Laura Pulliam, and Nicole Moore, who guided me through this entire project.

I want to thank my two most memorable mentors. Kim Beals may not realize it, but her guidance and mentorship through graduate school made me who I am. Thank you for building me up and believing in me. Also thanks to Juliet Mancino for her guidance years ago when I was a dietetic intern. You never gave me the answers but instead told me where to find them. Thank you for challenging me to be better.

Part I

Sport Nutrition for Today's Athletes

Chapter 1

Building a Champion

Champions do not decide their future. Champions decide their habits. Their habits decide their future.

This quote by Kevin Eastman is on a poster hanging in my office as a reminder of the critical role healthy habits play in creating a true champ. Children learn habits from a very young age, and they carry those habits into their teenage and adult years. I have heard comments such as this many times: "My child can eat whatever he wants because he's so active." However, nutrition is not just about weight; it's also about health. It's about building a strong body, immune system, and skeleton from the inside out. It's about developing healthy habits from a young age so that they stick with you throughout your life.

My daughter first played soccer at the local YMCA. At only four years old, the kids were being taught how to be young athletes—warm up and stretch, play, water break, play, water break. They would get so excited to run to the sidelines and retrieve their water bottles from their parents. I would sit on my lawn chair and listen to the parents complain that the coaches stopped the game when the kids did not need a water break. After all, many of them, including my daughter, were more focused on picking dandelions in the field than actually running after the ball. But they sure did get excited about their water breaks.

What many of the parents didn't recognize was that the kids were being taught a very important habit. They were learning that if you participate in sports and exercise, taking water breaks is important. The coaches were teaching them the habit of healthy hydration.

Teaching healthy habits from a very young age leads to adolescents and adults with healthy habits. It's the first step in building star athletes.

Given that you purchased a book on fueling youth athletes, you might assume that you'll be reading only about nutrition. But being a star athlete requires more than just having healthy eating habits. Winners realize that lifestyle plays

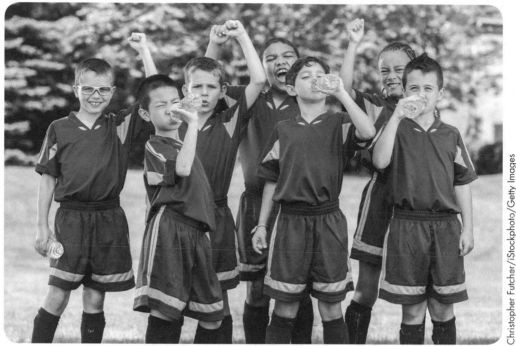

Christopher Futcher/iStockphoto/Getty Images

Healthy hydration habits should start at a very young age. Athletes who are taught to take water breaks every 15 minutes grow up to be teenage and adult athletes who understand and practice healthy hydration.

a critical role in athletic success. Physical training, sport nutrition and hydration, sleep, determination, attitude, commitment, and maturity all play roles in athletic achievement. Good genetics helps, too. In fact, having the entire package is what makes young athletes so attractive to scouting agents and coaches. Pushing children too far too soon can have negative consequences, both mentally and physically. We want to help them be the best, but young athletes are still children; we need to remember and respect that as we provide guidance.

Training and Teenage Development

If you watch young athletes compete, you have probably identified a few kids who have a natural talent for sports. They seem to have inherited all of the right genes to be star players. Without much effort, they seem to just get it. Although it is true that genetics plays a role in athletic talent, it is unlikely to deliver a championship title without some added effort. Proper physical training that is appropriate for the developmental age of the athlete is a critical piece.

My private practice, Nutrition CheckUp, is located within a facility that trains young athletes, so I see firsthand the extensive evaluation that happens when they train in the right environment. Jeremy Hoy, MS, CSSD, a strength and conditioning coach who specializes in long-term athletic development, has a formal procedure for determining whether a young athlete is ready for serious training. His process includes an evaluation of movement, fitness, and performance that he describes as follows:

> The evaluation is intentionally challenging to see if the athlete is willing to work hard and push through the struggle. It also gives us an opportunity to assess the athlete's coachability, or willingness to be coached and to listen. If an athlete can focus and pay attention and is willing to work through the evaluation (can take a realistic look at where he or she is on these tests) and doesn't quit, then the chances of integrating successfully into our training system is over 95 percent (personal communication).

Young athletes who are not showing signs of mental or physical maturity don't have to be barred from training. They just need more time to develop before they are pushed to the next level. These athletes should focus on other areas, such as developing proper sleep habits or building a solid sport nutrition plan.

Steve Reich, an NHLPA-certified agent with O2K Worldwide Management Group, acts as a family adviser for young athletes who plan to attend Division I hockey schools before playing professional hockey. He explained the following:

> What we look for in young guys are a high compete level on and off the ice, a strong work ethic, hockey sense, and an overall commitment to being the best athletes they can be (personal communication).

Winning lifestyle and personality characteristics come naturally to some young athletes and are often observed from a very young age. When the strong desire and commitment to succeed appear, it can be tempting to push them to train harder or eat differently to promote physical development. But children enter adolescence and puberty at varying ages. Exercising at any stage of maturity will make a person stronger, but significant muscular development won't happen until the body is ready. Well-trained coaches, trainers, and sport dietitians know how to work with younger athletes to evaluate and determine their readiness to advance to the next level. Parental support and understanding are also critical during these stages of life. Pushing too hard too soon can add to the stress of being a teen.

It is important to remember that children and teenagers are not mini-adults. The teenage brain processes information differently than the adult brain does, and the teenage body goes through extraordinary changes in development. A basic understanding of these differences can help youth athletes and those who guide them develop proper athletic training.

The Teenage Brain

Body changes are not the only changes teenagers experience; their brains are in the process of maturing as well. Adolescents sort out information differently than adults do because their decision-making and problem-solving skills are not fully developed. They don't spend much time considering how their current behavior will affect future outcomes, and they can be quickly persuaded by the wrong influences. Social networking sites, magazines, movies, television shows, and many other media sources have a daily influence on their eating behaviors. Parents, coaches, and trainers can play an important role in helping them separate the facts from the fads.

A basic understanding of teenagers' developmental changes helps parents and coaches discuss realistic expectations with young athletes. In the early developmental stages, adolescents focus on fitting in. As they progress through the teenage years, their worries about being normal continue, but they begin to move toward developing their own identities and forming relationships with peers. It is not until later adolescence that a firmer identity is formed. Table 1.1 provides an overview of cognitive development throughout adolescence.

The Teenage Body

Puberty is not a point in time but rather a process in which the body changes from that of a child to that of an adult. Children begin puberty at varying ages, and males and females face different struggles with their growing bodies. The changes that occur can affect how they look and feel about themselves, especially as they compare themselves to their teammates. Coaches and parents clearly notice the physical changes; they should be equally familiar with how those changes may affect feelings and performance.

Table 1.1 Psychosocial Processes and the Stages of Adolescent Development

	Early adolescence (ages 11-14)	Middle adolescence (ages 15-17)	Later adolescence (ages 18-21)
Emotionally related	Adjustment to a new body image, adaptation to emerging sexuality	Establishment of emotional separation from parents	Establishment of personal sense of identity, further separation from parents
Cognitively related	Concrete thinking, early moral concepts	Emergence of abstract thinking, expansion of verbal abilities and conventional morality, adjustment to increased school demands	Development of abstract, complex thinking; emergence of postconventional morality
Socially related	Strong peer effect	Increased health risk behaviors, sexual interest in peers, early vocational plans	Increased impulse control, emerging social autonomy, establishment of vocational capability

Adapted, by permission, from G.M. Ingersoll, 1992, Psychological and social development. In *Textbook of adolescent medicine*, edited by E.R. McAnarney, et al. (Philadelphia: Saunders), 92.

Fuel Focus

Tracy

Tracy, a 12-year-old volleyball player, was embarrassed when she went school shopping with her friends and re- alized that her pants size was much bigger than theirs. Her mom, Joan, called me to see if I could help. She ex- 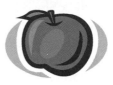 plained that Tracy plays volleyball and has always been on the heavier side, but recently she has started to gain more weight. Joan admitted that she had noticed and would tell Tracy that she needed to stop eating so much junk. Joan believed she was doing the right thing by bringing atten- tion to Tracy's food choices. She admitted that a fight often ensued when she criticized Tracy's diet. After the school shopping incident, Tracy was upset. She could not understand why her friends could eat whatever they wanted but be so much thinner than she was—after all, she was an ath-

lete. Tracy was entering the next stage of puberty, and her eating habits were catching up to her. At just 12 years old, Tracy was already feeling the pressure to go on a diet.

Joan was smart to schedule a nutrition consultation with me. Parents and coaches naturally want to help. But pointing out that bad food choices are caus- ing growing children to become overweight can put a strain on them and negatively affect par- ents' and coaches' relationships with them. Children need to feel loved and accepted, whether they are overweight, underweight, or at an ideal weight. Parents and coaches need to remember that body changes are normal and keep the conversation about eat- ing habits related to health and sport performance, not body im- age.

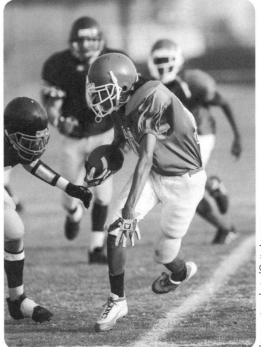

davepeetersphoto/Getty Images

Children hit puberty at various ages, and the changes that occur can affect not only how they look and feel but also how they perform at their sport.

As teenage girls go through puberty, they experience a fairly dramatic change in body fat and lean body mass. Throughout adolescence, average body fat levels increase from 16 to 27 percent, and lean body mass decreases slightly. Although normal, these changes are not always welcomed by young female athletes. Dramatic changes in body shape and size can lead to poor body image, low self-esteem, and disordered eating patterns. (See chapter 7 for more information on this.)

Males face different body composition changes during puberty than females do. They tend to gain lean body mass and decrease their body fat. The main hormone responsible for muscle growth during puberty is testosterone (also known as the sex hormone). Young male athletes usually welcome this rise in testosterone because it means building bigger muscles and becoming stronger. But males who enter puberty at a later age may feel discouraged as they are compared to their developing teammates. Those feelings may increase the temptation to try anabolic steroids and other supplements to increase muscle growth and development. Coaches, trainers, and parents can help young athletes understand the stages of change. They can reassure athletes that they

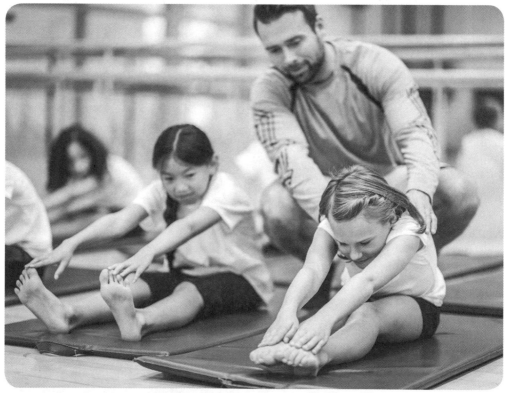

Christopher Futcher/Getty Images

Many aspects of athletic development should be taught before focusing on building muscle, such as the importance of stretching, practicing good form, coordination, and the importance of healthy foods and fluids.

Table 1.2 Tanner Stages of Development in Boys

	Development of external genitalia	Development of pubic hair	Linear growth in cm (in.) per year
Stage 1	Prepubertal.	Prepubertal; no pubic hair.	5-6 cm (2-2.4 in.)
Stage 2	Enlargement of scrotum and testes; scrotum skin reddens and changes in texture.	Sparse growth of hair at base of penis.	5-6 cm (2-2.4 in.)
Stage 3	Enlargement of penis (length at first); further growth of testes.	Darkening, coarsening, and curling; increase in amount.	7-8 cm (2.8-3 in.)
Stage 4	Increased size of penis with growth in breadth and development of glans; testes and scrotum larger, scrotum skin darker. Boys show a significant rise in circulating growth hormone levels at this stage (which is significantly later than in girls).	Hair resembles adult type but not spread to medial thighs.	10 cm (4 in.)
Stage 5	Adult genitalia.	Adult type and quantity spread to medial thighs.	No further height increase after ~17 years.

Adapted from W.A. Marshall and J.M. Tanner, 1970, "Variations in the pattern of pubertal changes in boys," *Archives of Diseases in Childhood* 45(239): 13-23.

can't force puberty, but they can focus on other aspects of athletic development. One way young athletes can help their bodies is by taking in proper foods and fluids.

The stages of development, also known as the Tanner stages, are more critical for determining energy needs and the ability to build muscle than is chronological age. Table 1.2 identifies the Tanner stages of development in boys; table 1.3 identifies the Tanner stages of development in girls.

As a parent or coach, you will not be able to evaluate the Tanner stage by the criteria in tables 1.2 and 1.3, so you will need a simpler approach. In addition to height changes, look for changes in skin (oilier, possibly resulting in pimples), body odor, body hair, and voice (deepening).

Table 1.3 Tanner Stages of Development in Girls

	Breast development	Development of pubic hair	Linear growth in cm (in.) per year
Stage 1	Prepubertal.	Prepubertal: no pubic hair.	5-6 cm (2-2.4 in.)
Stage 2	Breast bud stage with elevation of breast and papilla; enlargement of areola. Girls show a significant rise in circulating growth hormone levels at this stage, with the highest levels at stage 3-4).	Sparse growth of hair along labia.	7-8 cm (2.8-3 in.)
Stage 3	Further enlargement of breast and areola; no separation of their contour.	Pigmentation, coarsening, and curling with an increase in amount.	8 cm (3 in.)
Stage 4	Areola and papilla form a secondary mound above level of breast.	Hair resembles adult type but not spread to medial thighs.	7 cm (2.8 in.)
Stage 5	Mature stage; projection of papilla only, related to recession of areola.	Adult type and quantity, spread to medial thighs.	No further height increase after ~16 years.

Adapted from W.A. Marshall and J.M. Tanner, 1969, "Variations in pattern of pubertal changes in girls," *Archives of Diseases in Childhood* 44(235): 281-303.

Impact of Sport Nutrition

Sport nutrition has come a long way from when I was a young athlete. Back then, the phrase *sport nutrition* did not exist. Although the team headed to the local ice cream shop for a postgame celebration, it was not because we were attempting to help our muscles recover. In fact, that was the last thing on our minds. Today, young athletes are starting their sports earlier, and the impact on their growing bodies is more recognized. Sport nutrition is a hot topic and is proven to provide performance benefits for athletes of all ages.

Sport nutrition refers to the food and fluid needed to support the additional training and activity of an athlete. It includes not only the foods consumed before, during, and after a workout but also the additional nutrition needed day to day to support weekly training. Remember that the goal of the sport nutrition

Pressure on Today's Young Athletes

Youth athletics is not the same today as it was years ago. The popularity of organized sport continues to rise; an estimated 45 million U.S. children and adolescents participate in sports. Seventy-five percent of American families with school-aged children have at least one child in organized sports.

Today, children playing sports are dealing with greater pressure and more competition than children did years ago. Adolescent athletes report stressors related to both their sports and their lives in general; these stressors are listed in table 1.4.

In the right environment, youth sports provide a fun and rewarding opportunity to develop psychological well-being, establish friendships, and learn lifelong lessons to create a healthy and active lifestyle.

Table 1.4 Stressors Reported by Adolescent Athletes

Sport-related stressors	Organization stressors
Making physical or mental errors	Balancing schoolwork and sport training
Parent, teacher, and coach criticisms	Travel for sports
Pressure to perform	Day-to-day time management
Fear of injury	

Source: K.A. Tamminen, N.L. Holt, and P.R.E. Crocker, 2012, "Adolescent athletes: Psychosocial challenges and clinical concerns," *Current Opinion in Psychiatry* 25(4): 293-300.

plan is to support the athlete's training plan. In chapter 3 we cover the fuel needed for working muscles in more detail. Chapter 5 provides more specific information, including what to eat and when to eat to best support athletes in training.

Believe it or not, putting the plan in place is the most difficult part of sport nutrition. Even with the best intentions, young athletes may not have access to what they need or the ability to do what they need to do. A strong support system will help them get what they need. Sport dietitians can work with young athletes to create perfect meal plans for fueling their bodies during training, but if the athletes don't have someone to purchase the food and beverages, they won't be able to follow the plan. Part III of this book provides a play-by-play for creating a personal plan and for breaking down the barriers many families face in putting the plan into practice.

As I said at the beginning of this chapter, becoming a champion athlete is more than simply having good genes; it is more than pushing a motivated athlete to lift heavier weights or drink a protein shake after a workout. Building a champion athlete starts with encouraging healthy habits from a young age and understanding how the athlete thinks, grows, and develops. Now that you have a basic understanding of what it takes to build a champion, it is time to discover how nutrition influences growth, development, and sport performance.

Chapter 2

Day-to-Day Nutrition for Healthy Growth

Because I counsel young athletes, I work with a lot of parents and families. Most parents have very specific questions about fueling for sports. They want to know what to eat before an event, how much to drink during a game, and what the best meal is for recovery. Although these are all important questions that are addressed in this book, the foods that are eaten day to day play a much larger role in health and athletic performance. Adequate day-to-day nutrition is what supports healthy growth and development, boosts the immune system, and works to heal sport injuries.

This book begins with a discussion of the basics, because a solid diet foundation needs to be the number one priority. Athletes are unlikely to be the best they can be if they are sick or injured. A healthy, injury-free athlete equals a winning athlete. Just as athletes who participate in different sports have different energy requirements, growing children have different energy requirements from those of adults. Daily nutrition requirements vary based on developmental age, sex, body type, and body composition. Adding in a recovery meal, for example, when athletes' day-to-day nutritional requirements have not been met will do little to help them meet their athletic goals. Once daily nutritional needs are met, then the extra foods and fluids needed to support sport training become the focus.

Nutrition Basics

The body gets its energy from food, which should provide a variety of vitamins and minerals. Unfortunately, that is not always the case. Some foods provide the calories needed for growth but do not provide the nutrients needed for

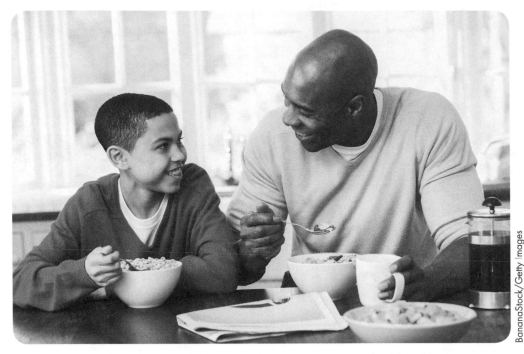

BananaStock/Getty Images

Adequate day to day nutrition is the first consideration in growing a healthy athlete.

supporting development. The result is usually an overweight yet undernourished body.

The best food supports the growth, development, and maintenance of muscles, bones, organs, skin, and blood to cleanse, oxygenate, and nourish all parts of the body. The day-to-day diet should provide adequate amounts of all six essential nutrients that the body requires to function properly: water, carbohydrate, protein, fat, vitamins, and minerals. Athletes should understand the role and function of each of the essential nutrients, and they should have a general understanding of how much they need of each. See figure 2.1 for each nutrient's role.

The essential nutrients are divided into three categories: macronutrients, micronutrients, and water. The macronutrients (carbohydrate, protein, and fat) supply the energy needed to fuel working muscles. For that reason, they are referred to as the energy-yielding nutrients. That energy is measured in calories. Vitamins and minerals (also called micronutrients) do not supply energy, but they are vital to life and needed for normal growth and development. Finally, water does not supply energy, but it is a component of all cells and is vital for life.

In addition to providing the nutrients vital for life, foods provide phytochemicals (i.e., compounds that give the foods classified as superfoods their super powers). Phytochemicals are believed to help protect against certain diseases. Aside from the potential health benefits, many phytonutrients may help reduce inflammation, thereby boosting immune function and improving focus and concentration, all things that help athletes perform well.

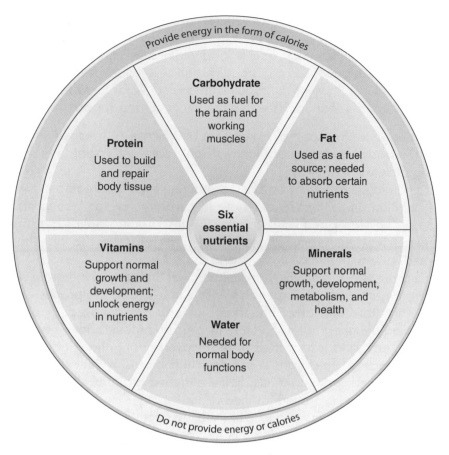

Figure 2.1 The six essential nutrients.

Let's talk a little more about each nutrient—how much you need and the role it plays in proper growth and development.

Carbohydrate

Our bodies use the carbohydrate we eat to provide energy. Carbohydrate is the preferred source of fuel for working muscles, and it supplies a steady source of energy to feed the brain and nervous system. Foods rich in carbohydrate are broken down in the body into glucose. Glucose can be used immediately or stored in the liver and muscles until it is needed.

Every gram of carbohydrate provides 4 calories, but that doesn't mean that all carbohydrates are created equal. They are divided into two categories, complex carbohydrates and simple carbohydrates, as follows:

- *Complex carbohydrates* are long chains of sugar units arranged to form starch or fiber. They are found in foods such as bread, cereal, rice, pasta, beans, starchy vegetables (such as corn and potatoes), and nonstarchy vegetables (such as green beans and broccoli). These foods provide energy along with a variety of vitamins, minerals, and phytonutrients.

- *Simple carbohydrates* include both single sugar units and linked pairs of sugar units. They include the sugar that is found naturally in foods (such as fruit, milk, milk products, and vegetables) as well as in foods with added sugar (such as candy, sugar-sweetened beverages, and many desserts). In general, foods with added sugar have fewer nutrients per calorie than foods with naturally occurring sugar.

Both categories of carbohydrate end up as glucose or fructose and can be used by the body for energy. If planned right, both are valuable fuel sources for young athletes.

In addition to categorizing carbohydrate into simple and complex, many of today's nutrition and fitness books refer to carbohydrate as good carbs and bad carbs. The term *good carbs* is used to describe those that are higher in fiber and rich in whole grains. The term *bad carbs* is used to describe those that are refined, or made with white flour and added sugar.

Whole grain refers to grains that contain all of the parts of the grain seed, or kernel (bran, germ, and endosperm). When whole grains are processed, some of the dietary fiber and other important nutrients are removed. A processed grain is called a refined grain. Some refined grain products have key nutrients, such as folic acid and iron, which were removed during the initial processing and added back in. These are called enriched grains. White rice and white bread are enriched grain products. Some enriched grain foods have extra nutrients added. These are called fortified grains.

The current U.S. recommended dietary allowance (RDA) of carbohydrate is a minimum of 130 grams per day, but that doesn't mean that is all you need. This RDA is based on its role as the primary energy source for the brain and not on the added activity of a young athlete. Athletes need to remember that carbohydrate provides the energy that fuels their activity, and their needs are higher than those of the average sedentary person.

The body's ability to store glucose in the liver and muscles is of critical importance, especially for athletes. Stored glucose, known as glycogen, is what feeds the brain and fuels the muscles, helping athletes to focus and keep going during prolonged activity. The amount of glycogen that muscles can store is influenced by training. A well-trained muscle can store more glycogen than an untrained muscle can. Even a well-trained athlete, however, has glycogen-storing limits. Once the body has enough carbohydrate to burn for energy and the muscle and liver are filled, the remaining glucose is stored as fat. As young athletes grow and develop, their ability to build muscle increases, as does their ability to store glycogen.

Protein

In the world of sport nutrition, the word *protein* conjures visions of shaker bottles and flexed muscles. But the protein we eat does much more than build, repair, and maintain muscles. Without protein, life would not exist. Hair, nails, skin, tendons, muscles, organs, immune systems, and the core of bones and teeth—all of these contain protein.

Eating Vegetarian or Vegan

Vegetarian and vegan diets are popular among youth athletes, especially females. Teenagers may decide to follow such a diet for a variety of reasons, including animal rights, religious convictions, or perceived health benefits. It might also be because friends are doing it. If your athlete decides to follow this type of eating style, it is important to find out why. Some do so for misguided reasons, such as weight control, which is not an appropriate use.

Following are four types of vegetarian diets:

- *Semi-vegetarian.* This type may allow all or certain animal products but only in small amounts.
- *Lacto-ovo vegetarian.* This type permits dairy and eggs but excludes red meat, fish, and fowl.
- *Lacto-vegetarian.* This type allows dairy (e.g., milk, cheese, and yogurt) but excludes eggs, red meat, fish, and fowl.
- *Vegan.* This type of diet excludes all animal products.

Even though we have these clear definitions, children and teenagers often create their own rules and guidelines. Many teenagers are quick to remove foods from their diet without considering the nutrients that they were getting from those foods. When food groups are eliminated, special consideration must be given to how those vitamins and minerals will be obtained. That's why understanding where we get our nutrients is so important.

Protein is made up of 20 amino acids, about half of which are essential, meaning that we have to get them from the foods we eat. Without these essential amino acids, the body cannot make the protein it needs to do its work. Like carbohydrate, protein provides 4 calories per gram, but not all dietary protein is created equal. We classify protein as complete, incomplete, or complementary, based on how many essential amino acids it contains, as follows:

- A *complete protein* is one that provides all of the essential amino acids. It is often referred to as a *high-quality protein.* Animal-based foods such as red meat, poultry, fish, milk, eggs, and cheese are considered complete protein sources.
- An *incomplete protein* source is one that is low in one or more of the essential amino acids. Legumes, nuts, seeds, grains, and vegetables are examples of incomplete protein sources.
- *Complementary proteins* are two or more incomplete protein sources that together provide adequate amounts of all the essential amino acids. Beans and rice are a good example of complementary proteins.

Rice is a poor source of certain essential amino acids, but those essential amino acids are found in higher amounts in beans. Likewise, beans contain lower amounts of other essential amino acids that can be found in larger amounts in rice. Together, these two foods provide adequate amounts of all the essential amino acids. They complement each other. Young athletes who restrict intake of animal products or follow a vegetarian or vegan diet need to understand this concept.

It is worth mentioning that coaches, parents, and young athletes are often drawn to protein supplements, such as powders and bars, to increase protein intake. On occasion, these products have a place in the diet, but getting protein from natural food sources is important. Foods that have protein are also packed with vitamins and minerals needed for growth and development. Too much reliance on supplemental protein can leave youth athletes short of other important nutrients.

Protein needs are described in terms of grams of protein per kilogram of body weight. Needs are the highest during the time of peak gain in height, which typically occurs between the ages of 11 and 14 for females and 15 and 18 for males. Like energy needs, protein needs during the adolescent years are related more to growth patterns than age. Protein is an essential part of an adolescent athletes' diet, but eating extra will not lead to greater muscle mass. Some excessive protein can be used for immediate energy, or it might be stored as fat.

Dietary Fat

Fat is an important nutrient and fuel source for youth athletes. Fat absorbs some nutrients, provides essential fatty acids, protects vital organs, and serves as an insulator to keep the body warm. It is also an important fuel source for adolescents. Dietary fat also contributes to feeling full and can make food taste better.

Although fat is essential for normal body function, some types of fat are healthier than others. The dietary fat in food is divided into four major categories: trans fat, saturated fat, monounsaturated fat, and polyunsaturated fat.

The so-called bad fats are trans fat and saturated fat. Together, they can raise LDL (bad) cholesterol in the body. Most saturated fat comes from animal products such as beef, lamb, pork, poultry with skin, butter, cream, cheese, and other higher-fat dairy products. It is also created artificially to make liquid oils more solid. *Trans* fat can be found in fried foods and baked goods such as pastries, pizza dough, pie crust, cookies, and crackers. Today, many fast-food establishments and restaurants have stopped using trans fat in their products, and the U.S. Food and Drug Administration (FDA) is considering banning its use in processed foods. Youth athletes should try to avoid trans fat. You can see whether a product contains trans fat by checking for partially hydrogenated oil on the ingredients list.

So-called good fats are the monounsaturated and polyunsaturated fats. When eaten in place of saturated fat and trans fat, they may help improve

Let's Learn About Omega-3 Fatty Acids

Omega-3 fatty acids are an important family of polyunsaturated fat. There are three main types. Eicosapentaenoic acid (EPA) and docosahexaenoic acid (DHA) come mainly from fish. Alpha-linolenic acid (ALA) is found in some vegetable oils, walnuts, flaxseeds and flaxseed oil, leafy vegetables, and tofu (there are trace amounts in other foods). ALA is the most common omega-3 fatty acid in the Western diet, but it is different from EPA and ALA. ALA must be converted to EPA and DHA in the body, but the conversion is very limited. It is unlikely that anyone could eat enough walnuts or flaxseed to reap the benefits of omega-3. To consume adequate amounts of omega-3 fatty acids through food, you need to include fatty fish as part of your meal plan a few days a week. See table 2.1 for food sources of omega-3 fatty acids.

The data to support the importance of omega-3 fatty acids for the treatment of chronic diseases in adults are well established. It is also well researched as a way to treat attention-deficit/hyperactivity disorder (ADHD), autism, depression, and other health conditions. With so much interest in omega-3 fatty acids, and so few people eating enough fish, the marketing and sale of omega-3 supplements have skyrocketed. And they have reached into the sport performance world. For more information on the use of omega-3 in supplement form, see chapter 6.

Table 2.1　Food Sources of Omega-3 Fatty Acids

Food*	EPA (g)	DHA (g)
Mackerel, Atlantic, raw	0.90	1.40
Salmon, Chinook, raw	1.01	0.094
Herring, Atlantic, raw	0.69	1.46
Anchovy, canned in oil, drained solids	0.76	1.29
Salmon, sockeye, raw	0.35	0.68
Salmon, Atlantic, wild, raw	0.32	1.12
Salmon, canned, pink, total can contents	0.32	0.67
Tuna, white, canned in water, drained	0.23	0.63
Salmon, Chinook, smoked (lox)	0.18	0.27
Swordfish, raw	0.11	0.65
Tuna, light, canned in oil, drained	0.03	0.10
Egg, whole, cooked, hard boiled	0.00	0.04

*Based on a 100 g, or 3.5 oz, serving.

Source: US Department of Agriculture, Agricultural Research Service, Nutrient Data Laboratory. USDA National Nutrient Database for Standard Reference.

blood cholesterol levels. They are mainly found in fatty fish, nuts, seeds, avocados, and olives.

At 9 calories per gram, fat provides more calories than carbohydrate and protein and is therefore a very dense energy source. The *Dietary Guidelines for Americans* recommends that growing teenagers consume 25 to 35 percent of their total calories in the form of fat (U.S. Department of Health and Human Services and U.S. Department of Agriculture, 2015). There are no specific guidelines for athletes; some require more fat than others do. Dietary fat should never be eliminated from an athlete's eating plan, even if the goal is to decrease body fat. The first focus is to get adequate amounts of carbohydrate and protein. The amount of fat will vary based on the athlete's body composition, goals, and total energy needs. Chapter 8 walks you through calculating the macronutrient requirements for meeting specific goals.

Water

There is a lot to talk about when it comes to fluids. The body needs more water each day than any other nutrient. Without it, we can survive only a few days. Water transports nutrients throughout the body and removes the waste products of metabolism. It also functions as a lubricant, as part of saliva and the fluid surrounding the joints. One of the most important functions of water is to cool the body. Working muscles generate heat, which raises body temperature. If the fluid lost in sweat is not replaced, dehydration can occur.

Children who have not reached puberty are at even higher risk for overheating than adolescents who have. For one, children have a lower sweating capacity than adults, leaving them less effective at dissipating excess body heat. They also take longer to adjust to warmer temperatures.

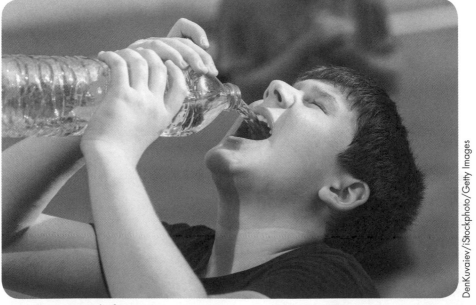

DenKuvaiev/iStockphoto/Getty Images

Water is the most vital of nutrients.

Table 2.2   Dietary Reference Intakes for Water

	Males	Females
Ages 9-13	2.4 liters = 10 cups	2.1 liters = 9 cups
Ages 14-18	3.3 liters = 14 cups	2.3 liters = 10 cups

Healthy adolescents can generally regulate their fluid intake and avoid dehydration, but active young athletes need to pay close attention. Chapter 3 addresses the specifics of the extra fluids needed to support activity, body composition, and performance goals.

You might have heard that you need to drink eight glasses of water a day. I believe you need at least that much. Table 2.2 shows the dietary reference intakes (DRIs) for water (Institute of Medicine, 2006).

If you are far from drinking 14 cups of water a day, do not worry. That recommendation includes drinking water, water in other beverages, and the water you get from foods. Athletes, however, need more water than sedentary people do, to replace fluid losses through sweat. Chapter 3 provides more specific recommendations.

Vitamins and Minerals

Vitamins and minerals, also known as micronutrients, do not provide energy, but many of them are necessary to unlock the energy in carbohydrate, protein, and fat. Although we need them only in small amounts, they keep the body working properly and protect it from illness.

Vitamins are divided into two categories, water soluble and fat soluble. Because water-soluble vitamins (e.g., vitamin C and all of the B vitamins) dissolve in water, we cannot store them in water. Any amount over what is needed by the body is excreted in urine. Fat-soluble vitamins (vitamins A, D, E, and K) do not dissolve in water and are stored in the liver and in fat cells. To learn the exact amount you need of each vitamin and mineral, see table 2.4 later in this chapter.

But, remember, young athletes eat food, not nutrients. One of the main reasons registered dietitians encourage the consumption of a variety of foods is to make sure people eat a variety of nutrients.

Tools to Guide Smart Eating

During adolescence, significant growth and development occur, resulting in increased nutritional needs. In fact, nutrient needs during adolescence are higher than during any other time in life. Adequate nutrition is the key to reaching growth potential. Until puberty, nutrient needs for males and females are similar, but once puberty hits, the changes in body composition create a need for sex-specific recommendations.

Ruth

Ruth, a 16-year-old female runner, came to see me complaining of fatigue. After she had been following a vegetarian diet for almost three months, her mom became concerned that she was not eating enough. Before discussing the foods Ruth was eating, I wanted to understand why she had decided to follow this type of eating plan.

Ruth explained that she decided to follow a vegetarian diet because she did not like the way animals were treated. She also believed that a vegetarian diet was better for her body. Although Ruth's perception of animal welfare was not completely accurate, I respected her decision to follow the diet. As with many youth athletes, Ruth's vegetarian choices did not fit one of the preceding types. She referred to herself as a vegan, but she did eat salmon and other fatty fish, foods she perceived as healthy. She avoided most dairy products and eggs, but she did allow herself Greek yogurt.

Ruth made one classic mistake when starting her modified vegan diet. She focused on the foods she wanted to eliminate rather than consider the foods she would have to start eating to make up for the nutrients lost. A vegetarian diet can be a very healthy diet if carefully planned. Because it excludes certain foods, athletes can struggle to get enough protein as well as certain vitamins and minerals. The more restrictive the diet is, the more thought that must go into planning it. Nutrients of the most concern are protein, calcium, vitamin D, iron, zinc, and vitamin B_{12}.

A vegetarian who eats dairy, eggs, and fish should have no problem getting enough high-quality protein. Still, some of the protein will come from incomplete protein sources. A vegan diet is the most restrictive and requires the most consideration. Because vitamin B_{12} is found almost exclusively in animal products, vegan athletes are at risk of falling short in that vitamin.

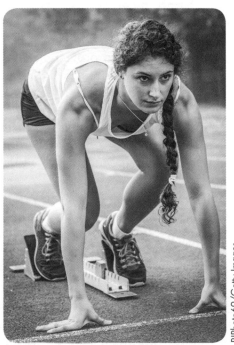

Young athletes who follow vegetarian or vegan diets must take special care in meal planning to meet their nutritional needs.

PJPhoto69/Getty Images

Vegans rely solely on plant-based protein sources to meet their needs. That means extra consideration is needed when selecting carbohydrate sources. All of the essential amino acids can be supplied by a variety of plant-based protein sources such as nuts, seeds, beans, whole grains, and soy foods.

In addition, I suggest that vegan athletes supplement their diets with nutritional yeast, which is rich in B vitamins, including B_{12}. It has a cheesy flavor and can be sprinkled on baked potatoes, popcorn, and vegetables or used as a condiment on other foods. It also tastes good as an ingredient in salad dressing.

Through careful planning and consideration, vegetarian and vegan athletes can build an adequate sport nutrition plan to meet their goals.

A few tools can help us eat right. One is the *Dietary Guidelines for Americans 2015-2020*. The *Dietary Guidelines* forms the basis of U.S. federal nutrition policy, education, outreach, and food assistance programs used by consumers, industry, nutrition educators, and health professionals. All federal dietary guidance for the public is required to be consistent with the *Dietary Guidelines*, which provides a scientific basis from which the government can speak in a consistent and uniform manner. In general, the *Dietary Guidelines* encourage individuals to eat a healthful diet—one that focuses on foods and beverages that help achieve and maintain a healthy weight, promote health, and prevent chronic disease (U.S. Department of Health and Human Services and U.S. Department of Agriculture, 2015). For more information, visit www.health.gov/dietaryguidelines.

Another tool, MyPlate, as shown in figure 2.2, is a practical way to put the *Dietary Guidelines* into practice. This food icon, created by the U.S. government, serves as a reminder to make good food choices. It illustrates the five food groups that form the foundation of a healthy diet. The food groups that make up the plate may be the same for all growing adolescents, although the amount of food will differ. For example, a 13-year-old gymnast and a 17-year-old linebacker can both use the plate to guide their food choices, but the linebacker may need to eat double the amount of food to meet his nutritional needs. The website www.choosemyplate.gov provides more information, including tips and tools for calculating individual nutrition needs and food portion sizes.

MyPlate provides guidance for building a healthy diet, but the dietary reference intakes (DRIs) provide the best estimate of each nutrient for children and adolescents. They take into account individual factors such as age and sex, and consider the growth and development that happens during adolescence (see table 2.4).

Think Before You Eliminate

Before you decide to avoid an entire food group, take some time to consider the nutrients you could be limiting in your diet. Eliminating a food group can make it hard to reach your recommended intake of the vitamins or minerals that food group provides. For example, the dairy group is an easy way to get calcium and vitamin D in your diet. By avoiding milk, cheese, and yogurt, you are not just limiting dairy foods; you are limiting your ability to take in the vital nutrients those foods provide. It is true that many vitamins and minerals can be found across food groups, but that is not the case for all of them. Before you eliminate a food group, consider how you will get those nutrients from other foods. Table 2.3 provides examples of the nutrients you can expect to obtain from each food group.

Although all vitamins and minerals are essential and should be included in every diet, some deserve more attention throughout the adolescent years. Chapter 3 includes a discussion of the ones that play a key role in producing energy, preventing fatigue, ensuring bone health, and developing muscles.

Table 2.3   Nutrients in Each Food Group

Vegetables	Potassium, dietary fiber, folate (folic acid), vitamin A, vitamin C
Grains	Dietary fiber, several B vitamins (thiamin, riboflavin, niacin, folate), minerals (iron, magnesium, selenium)
Fruits	Potassium, dietary fiber, vitamin C, folate (folic acid)
Protein	Protein, B vitamins (niacin, thiamin, riboflavin, B_6), vitamin E, iron, zinc, magnesium
Dairy	Protein, calcium, vitamin D, potassium

Even with tools to guide us, the amount of food that adolescents need can vary significantly depending on their stage of maturation and physical activity level. Chapter 8 explains how to create a personal eating plan using these tools and how to adjust a plan based on the energy demands of particular sports and training schedules.

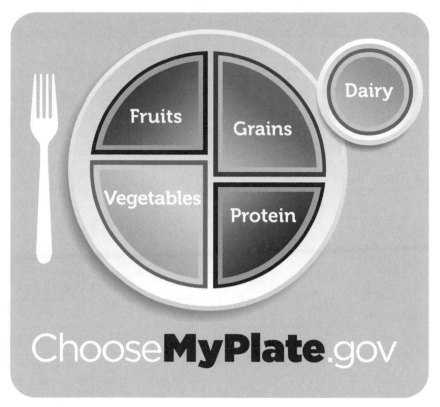

Figure 2.2 MyPlate.
USDA Center for Nutrition Policy and Promotion

Parents and caretakers play an enormous role in setting up growing athletes for eating success. Children learn most of their eating habits at home, and they carry what they learn throughout adolescence and into adulthood. As they get older, friends begin to have a larger influence. Building healthy habits, especially eating and hydration habits, is important from a very young age. Teenagers who have grown up with healthy day-to-day eating habits will be ahead of the game when it comes to the next phase of building a training plan. They are ready to add the fluids and fuel needed for improving their sport performance.

Table 2.4 Dietary Reference Intakes for Children and Adolescents

	Children		Males		Females	
	1-3 years	4-8 years	9-13 years	14-18 years	9-13 years	14-18 years
Calcium (mg/d)	700	1,000	1,300	1,300	1,300	1,300
Carbohydrate (g/d)	130	130	130	130	130	130
Protein (g/d[a])	13	19	34	52	34	46
Vitamin A (µg/d)[a]	300	400	600	900	600	700
Vitamin C (mg/d)	15	25	45	75	45	65
Vitamin D (IU/d)	600	600	600	600	600	600
Vitamin E (mg/d)[b]	6	7	11	15	11	15
Thiamin (mg/d)	0.5	0.6	0.9	1.2	0.9	1.0
Riboflavin (mg/d)	0.5	0.6	0.9	1.3	0.9	1.0
Niacin (mg/d)[c]	6	8	12	16	12	14
Vitamin B_6 (mg/d)	0.5	0.6	1.0	1.3	1.0	1.2
Folate (µg/d)[d]	150	200	300	400	300	400
Vitamin B_{12} (µg/d)	0.9	1.2	1.8	2.4	1.8	2.4
Copper (µg/d)	340	440	700	890	700	890
Iodine (µg/d)	65	65	73	95	73	95
Iron (mg/d)	7	10	8	11	8	15
Magnesium (mg/d)	80	130	240	410	240	360
Molybdenum (µg/d)	17	22	34	43	34	43
Phosphorus (mg/d)	460	500	1,250	1,250	1,250	1,250
Selenium (µg/d)	20	30	40	55	40	55
Zinc (mg/d)	3	5	8	11	8	9

For detailed notes pertaining to the DRI values, visit the individual reports and tables at https://ods.od.nih.gov/Health_Information/Dietary_Reference_Intakes.aspx

Data from documents available through the National Institutes of Health Office of Dietary Supplements, n.d., Nutrient recommendations: Dietary reference intakes (DRI). [Online]. Available: https://ods.od.nih.gov/Health_Information/Dietary_Reference_Intakes.aspx [August 31, 2016]. Documents issued by the Food and Nutrition Board and the Institute of Medicine, National Academy of Sciences.

Part II

Nutrition Needs for Sports and Individual Goals

Chapter 3

Fueling and Hydrating for Sport

The extraordinary growth and development that occur during the adolescent years can make estimating total energy needs difficult. Add to that the energy expenditure from sport participation, and the task can be quite a challenge. Determining how much more food and fluid an athlete needs depends on many factors. Most important, the additional nutritional considerations to meet those goals should be considered only after what is needed for adequate growth and development is reached. This chapter discusses fueling above and beyond young athletes' basic needs.

Fuel for Active Youth

Every athlete has unique goals. A young baseball player may want to lose weight to improve his speed. A football player may be looking to gain weight to improve his strength. A skater may want help to decrease fatigue. A hockey player may require strategies for maintaining weight during the season.

In my private practice, the initial appointment involves an interview. I always ask my clients to tell me four things they believe are wrong with their diet. One that usually makes the list is inconsistency—eating a lot of food one day and little food on another day. Those who notice this the most are generally the ones looking to gain weight.

Adolescents are often shocked when I say, "That is totally normal." I go on to explain that as they grow, their nutritional needs grow with them. During a growth spurt, appetite can increase significantly. When the growth spurt slows down, so does the appetite. All growing teenagers need enough food for growth, development, activity, and health; youth athletes simply need more. They don't require more of every vitamin and mineral, but they do require more of the macronutrients that provide energy. They also need to pay special attention to certain micronutrients, especially those involved in providing energy, preventing fatigue, ensuring bone health, and developing muscles. This section addresses the fuel and nutrients needed for working muscles.

Energy Needs of Youth Athletes

How many calories do growing athletes need? That might seem like a simple question, but a lot goes into calculating their total energy needs. As discussed in chapter 1, boys and girls enter puberty at different ages, which means that the need for increased energy to support their linear growth and changes in body composition and bone mass comes at different ages. Even after puberty, athletes come in all shapes and sizes. And it doesn't stop there. Add physical training, sport practice, and competitions, and the result is highly variable energy needs. All of these variables must be considered when calculating the foods and fluids needed for supporting a youth athlete's training program.

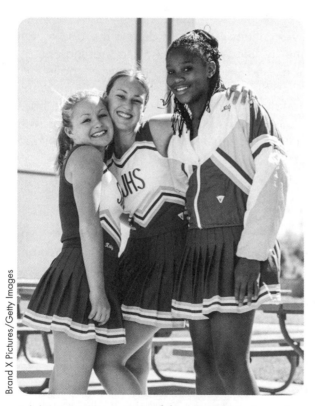

Brand X Pictures/Getty Images

I use the term *youth athlete* to refer to children and teenagers up to age 18 who participate in sports. The 10-year-old who plays recreational baseball twice a week, the 9-year-old competitive gymnast who practices 13 hours a week, and the 17-year-old hockey player who skates on two competitive teams—all of these fall under this umbrella term. In reality, the sport experiences of youth athletes vary significantly, based on the intensity and competitive nature of the sport, intensity of the training, and length of the season. In addition, many youth athletes participate on multiple teams or traveling teams or play multiple sports. All of this means that one young athlete may need only an additional 200 calories per day to support his activity, whereas another may need an additional 1,500 calories per day.

Adolescent athletes, even of the same chronological age, come in all shapes and sizes. When determining nutrition needs, developmental age must be considered in addition to individual goals.

For adult athletes, formulas have been developed to estimate the number of calories burned when participating in different sports and at different intensities. But that's not the case for youth athletes. Scientific studies have attempted to show energy expenditure, but because no validated tools are available, different approaches have been used in different studies. For example, one study estimated energy expenditure to be as high as 4,000 calories in adolescent male speedskaters (Ekelund, 2002). Using a different measuring technique, adolescent female judokas were estimated to expend approximately 2,600 calories (Boisseau, 2005). In male distance runners, daily energy expenditure was estimated to be about 3,600 calories, whereas in females it was about 2,500 calories (Eisenmann, 2007). This suggests that even within the same sport, the sex of the athlete has a significant influence on energy expenditure.

Although we do not have reliable evidence to prove it, there is reason to assume that youth athletes expend more calories than adult athletes do during exercise. We do know that children have a higher resting energy expenditure than adults do. Simply stated, per kilogram of body mass, children burn more calories at rest than adults do. The differences in their stride and muscle contractions likely play a role. Children are just less efficient in their movements, which results in a higher calorie demand. As they become better trained in their sports, their energy demands likely decrease.

The total energy expenditure for youth athletes has traditionally been evaluated based on physical activity levels (PAL) and resting energy expenditure (REE), but validated PAL recommendations are available only for adults (for estimated PAL recommendations in youth see table 8.6). The United Nations University (UNU), World Health Organization (WHO), and Food and Agriculture Organization of the United Nations (FAO) (2004) suggested PAL values for children and adolescents performing light to moderate activity, but not for competitive athletes. Researchers calculated the energy expenditure in 64 athletes ages 12 to 18 performing various sports and observed that the PAL range was somewhat higher (1.75 to 2.05) than UNU, WHO, and FAO suggested (1.5 to 1.85) for active adolescents (Carlsohn et al., 2011). Until we have a validated tool for calculating the energy needs of competitive adolescent athletes, we can use the PAL estimates as a starting point and then make adjustments as needed.

The estimated energy requirements (EER) for children and adolescents are based on energy expenditure, requirements for growth, and level of physical activity. Table 3.1 provides examples of the number of calories youth athletes may need based on age, height, weight, and activity level. Although a given athlete's age, height, and weight are unlikely to perfectly align with the examples, the chart can be used in estimating energy needs. Remember that significant variability for both males and females is likely as a result of variations in growth rate and the amount of time they spend in physical training, practice, and events. The DRIs are based on the chronological, not the developmental, age of the athlete, so using a combination approach to determining energy requirements in youth athletes is often necessary.

Table 3.1 Examples of EER (Calories) for Males and Females Ages 10 to 18

	Age	Reference weight (lb/kg)	Reference height (in./cm)	Sedentary PAL[1]	Low active PAL[2]	Active PAL[3]	Very active PAL[4]
Male	10	70/32	55/140	1,605	1,879	2,154	2,492
	12	90/41	58/147	1,793	2,108	2,423	2,810
	14	130/59	65/165	2,316	2,716	3,114	3,601
	16	150/68	69/175	2,527	2,969	3,412	3,956
	18	170/77	71/180	2,692	3,172	3,652	4,243
Female	10	70/32	55/140	1,475	1,734	1,978	2,384
	12	90/41	60/152	1,623	1,916	2,191	2,649
	14	105/48	62/157	1,677	1,987	2,281	2,768
	16	120/54	63/160	1,707	2,033	2,339	2,849
	18	130/59	66/168	1,763	2,108	2,431	2,970

[1]Rare in children.

[2]Less than 1 hour/day of activity.

[3]Approximately 1 hour/day of activity.

[4]More than 1 hour/day of activity.

Data based on calculations from J. Otten, J.P. Hellwig, and L.D. Meyers for Institute of Medicine of the National Academies, 2006, *Dietary Reference Intakes: The essential guide to nutrient requirements* (Washington, DC: National Academies Press), 82.

Use table 3.1 to help you estimate your own needs; then keep that number handy to record later in figure 8.5, My Daily Nutrient Needs.

Energy Guidelines for Youth Athletes

Extra activity requires extra calories, but loading up on pizza and chicken wings is not the answer. Some fuels are more beneficial than others. Let's talk about where the extra energy should come from to properly fuel working muscles.

Carbohydrate for Working Muscles

Carbohydrates, even the simple ones, are more complex than you may realize. Both simple and complex carbohydrates can add value to an athlete's performance, but the amount and the timing should be carefully considered. Complex carbohydrates are digested slowly and should make up the majority of a youth athlete's diet. They provide a steady source of energy throughout the day. The majority of the extra calories that a youth athlete needs should come from complex carbohydrates.

Simple carbohydrates digest quickly, thereby providing a great source of fuel when energy is needed quickly, such as immediately before an event, during an event, or between competitions. Both simple and complex carbo-hydrates are broken down into glucose for immediate energy or stored in the muscle and liver as glycogen for later use.

Carbohydrate provides the most efficient fuel for working muscles and can either greatly help or hinder progress. That's because the muscles are limited in the amount of carbohydrate they can store as glycogen. When muscle glycogen stores are used up, athletes have less energy, causing them to lose focus and decreasing their intensity and the quality of their performance. Injury surveys in U.S. youth soccer and the English Football Association showed that nearly 25 percent of all injuries occur in the last 15 to 20 minutes of games, when fatigue kicks in. This is also when the body becomes depleted of critical carbohydrate stores, which fuel the working brain and muscles. As they get tired, athletes lose concentration and put less focus into maintaining proper form. They become both mentally and physically drained.

Eating adequate amounts of carbohydrate has an additional benefit. It spares the breakdown of protein. This is especially important for youth athletes trying to gain weight and build muscle mass. When enough total calories are consumed, and the right amount is supplied as carbohydrate, protein can be used for what it is intended (growth and repair) rather than be broken down for energy.

How much additional carbohydrate to consume depends not only on the developmental age of the athlete but also on the type, intensity, and duration of training as well as the overall performance or body composition goal. As grow-ing athletes enter puberty and experience growth spurts, their carbohydrate intake needs to increase. The higher the total caloric needs are, the higher the carbohydrate intake must be. The goal must be considered when determining carbohydrate needs (e.g., improve performance, gain muscle, decrease body fat). All of these factors influence fuel choice and should be taken into consid-eration.

Fat for Working Muscles

Carbohydrate is known to provide the best fuel for working muscles, but fat is also a valuable fuel source during activity, especially in young athletes. Chil-dren have higher fat oxidation rates than adults have, suggesting that fat is a very valuable fuel during prolonged activity.

Both carbohydrate and fat are important for youth athletes, but which is the best source of energy still depends on the type, intensity, and duration of the activity. Fat requires oxygen to burn. When intensity is high, muscles have less oxygen and thus are unable to burn fat as efficiently. The body relies on the glycogen in muscles for brief, intense activities, such as sprinting and jumping; therefore, it is a valuable fuel in sports that require repeated bursts of energy, such as basketball, football, and volleyball. Because glycogen is used very quickly in intense activity, to make it through a game without running out of steam, athletes should start with glycogen-filled muscles. They may also need to take in additional fuel during a long game. This is where simple carbohydrates, such as those found in sport drinks, have an important role. Because simple sugars digest quickly, they can be used as an immediate energy source, providing additional fuel to keep energy levels high throughout a training session or event.

As the intensity of a sport decreases and the body has more oxygen available, such as during long-distance running or cycling, more fat can be used as energy. These endurance sports require a combination of glycogen and fat for energy.

Fat plays a very important role in the body, but too much or too little can negatively affect body composition and performance. If you recall from chapter 2, dietary fat is more nutrient dense than carbohydrate and protein; therefore, it contributes quite a bit more calories. Consuming too little fat can result in weight loss beyond what is optimal for athletic performance. Consuming too much fat can cause an increase in body fat, also leading to impaired performance. Athletes who want to gain weight may believe it is wise to eat higher-fat foods for the extra calories. This is not necessarily the best plan. Eating high-fat meals can decrease hunger, resulting in a lower consumption of the nutrients needed for proper growth and development. There is a right way and a wrong way to adjust body composition. Chapter 4 discusses how to manipulate nutrition to meet body composition goals.

Protein for Working Muscles

When it comes to sport nutrition, protein may be the most misunderstood nutrient. Yes, protein is needed to build muscle. But simply eating more protein will not increase muscle mass. The only way to build muscle mass is to put muscles to work and to eat an adequate amount of protein to support their repair and growth.

As with carbohydrate, youth athletes have a greater protein requirement than their nonathletic counterparts, but that does not mean more is better. In fact, consuming too much protein may get in the way of achieving performance goals. Protein guidelines exist for adult athletes, but requirements for youth athletes are not as easy to assess. Although many studies suggest that young athletes require more protein than their nonactive peers, the specific requirement may vary based on developmental stage, growth spurts, volume of training, and energy restriction for those in weight-class sports. Recommendations range from 1.0 to 1.8 grams per kilogram of body weight. A study of 14-year-old adolescent male soccer players suggested an RDA of 1.4 grams per kilogram of body weight per day (Boisseau et al., 2007).

In adults, protein recommendations for endurance athletes are 1.2 to 1.4 grams per kilogram of body weight; for power and strength athletes, 1.2 to 1.7. These amounts are expected to be appropriate for young athletes (children and adolescents) as well.

Following is the formula for determining a daily range of protein needs for a youth athlete:

$$\text{_____ weight in kg} \times 1.2 = \text{_____ g}$$

and

$$\text{_____ weight in kg} \times 1.7 = \text{_____ g}$$

For example, Jay is a 14-year-old male hockey player who weighs 140 pounds (64 kg). Using this calculation, his daily protein needs would be 77 to 109 grams per day, calculated like this:

$$64 \text{ kg} \times 1.2 = 77 \text{ g}$$

and

$$64 \text{ kg} \times 1.7 = 109 \text{ g}$$

Athletes who follow lower-calorie diets may have higher protein requirements. That is because when the body is not supplied with a sufficient amount of carbohydrate, some protein is converted and used for energy rather than muscle building. As a sport dietitian, I receive a lot of questions from youth athletes about which supplements they should take to increase protein in their diets. But even with their increased needs, most young athletes are getting more than enough protein without having to rely on supplementation. It is smart to get protein from foods rather than supplements. Whole-food sources of protein provide other beneficial nutrients as well. Many protein foods come packed with zinc, iron, magnesium, calcium, omega-3 fatty acids, B vitamins, vitamin E, and vitamin D.

Rather than worry about eating more protein, it is wise to focus on *when* to eat protein. Eating too much protein at one meal can create a feeling of fullness, resulting in consuming too few calories from other needed macronutrients. Eating too little protein can lead to muscle protein breakdown or prevent the development of new muscle tissue. Spreading protein intake equally over the course of the day may improve efficiency, optimize muscle protein synthesis, and enhance performance.

The meal plans in tables 3.2 and 3.3 both provide about 3,400 calories and 150 grams of protein, but in table 3.2, the protein intake is not evenly distributed. Very little is consumed during the breakfast and snack meals, whereas lunch and dinner have more than enough. Table 3.3 shows how to eat a better variety of foods so that protein intake is evenly distributed across the day.

Table 3.2 Unbalanced Daily Protein Distribution

Meal	Food items	Total protein
Breakfast	2 toaster pastries; 4 oz apple juice; banana	6 g
Lunch	2 turkey and cheese sandwiches on whole-wheat bread with mustard; tortilla chips with salsa; 12 oz milk	60 g
After-school snack	¼ cup peanuts, water	9 g
Dinner	2 grilled chicken breast sandwiches; 2 oz French fries; ketchup; 1 cup milk	72 g
Evening snack	2 oz pretzels; 8 oz apple juice	<1 g
	Total calories = ~3,400	Total protein = ~150 g

1 ounce solid = 30 grams; 8 ounces liquid = 240 ml.

Table 3.3 Optimized Daily Protein Distribution

Meal	Food items	Total protein
Breakfast	8 oz skim milk; 2 frozen waffles with syrup; banana; 2 turkey sausage links	32 g
Midmorning snack	8 oz skim milk; 2 granola bars; 1 oz Swiss cheese	17 g
Lunch	2 peanut butter and jelly sandwiches; 2 oz tortilla chips with salsa; water	32 g
After-school snack	8 oz Greek yogurt; 1/2 cup blueberries; 0.5 oz almonds	18 g
Dinner	1 grilled chicken sandwich; 1 oz French Fries; 1/2 cup mixed fruit; salad with raw vegetables and Italian dressing	34 g
Evening snack	Hard-boiled egg; 1 oz pretzels; 8 oz chocolate milk	17 grams
	Total calories = ~3,400	Total protein = ~150 g

1 ounce solid = 30 grams; 8 ounces liquid = 240 ml.

How much additional protein and when to consume it depend on the body composition goals of the athlete. As a rule, athletes can aim to eat 20 to 30 grams of protein at each meal and 10 to 20 grams at mini-meals and snacks. Females and those with lower protein requirements should stay on the lower end; males or those with higher protein requirements should aim for the higher end. We discuss protein's role in altering body composition in chapter 4. Chapter 8 explains how to create a meal plan with just enough protein to reach your personal goal.

Vitamins and Minerals for Active Youth

Conveniently, the vitamins and minerals needed for general health also play a role in building, maintaining, and supporting a body built to perform. Youth athletes do not require more vitamins or minerals than their nonathletic peers, but the consequences of insufficient intakes are likely to be more acute. Meeting the daily recommended requirements of each of them is important, but when it comes to youth athletes, a few of them require the spotlight. Let's take a look.

Fuel Focus

Jessica

Jessica is a 14-year-old speedskater suffering from multiple ankle fractures. Her orthopedic surgeon suggested that she see a registered dietitian to assess her nutritional intake.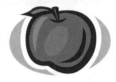

Jessica and her mom came to see me to evaluate her diet. Jessica was on crutches at the time. Both of her parents were very involved. They packed school lunches for her daily, prepared home-cooked meals, and supported the extra foods and fluids needed to support her active lifestyle. Although they took the advice of the surgeon and brought Jessica to see me, they believed that her diet was good.

While reviewing Jessica's food journal, I immediately noticed gaps in her nutrition. Jessica had very few sources of calcium or vitamin D in her diet; she did not drink milk, consumed yogurt only on occasion, and avoided cheese. Her diet was adequate in total energy, and her macronutrient distribution was spot-on. However, because certain critical nutrients were lacking, her performance and training were being jeopardized. In addition, as a skater, Jessica's training was indoors so she had minimal exposure to the sun.

Jessica was on board with doing whatever she needed to do to make her body stronger. Together, we created a meal plan that was adequate not only in total calories and macronutrients but also in vitamins and minerals. We reviewed the importance of these nutrients and the foods she could swap in her plan so that she continued to get them without eating the same foods every day.

Jessica went on her way. Months later, I received an e-mail from her mom letting me know that she was healed and doing great. She had also shaved an entire minute off her skating time.

Iron

In this book, I will not be able to say enough about the importance of iron. All parents, athletes, and coaches should be concerned about iron intake. Inadequate dietary iron intake may lie silent for weeks, months, even years, but the storm will come. When it does, it takes a while to reverse the symptoms.

Worldwide, iron deficiency it is the most common nutrient deficiency, and it is a significant concern for teenagers, especially girls. There is an increased need for iron during the adolescent years for both sexes, but for different reasons. Both girls and boys need more iron at this time to develop extra lean body mass, but girls also need more iron to support menstruation. If you consider the symptoms of deficiency, it becomes clear why iron is so important for athletes.

Iron is part of the protein hemoglobin, which carries oxygen in the blood, and part of the protein myoglobin in muscles, making oxygen available for muscle contraction. It helps these two proteins hold and carry oxygen and then release it. Iron depletion does not occur overnight; it results when iron intake is inadequate day after day, week after week. Inadequate iron intake will progress to iron deficiency and then to iron-deficiency anemia.

The early symptoms of iron deficiency include thinking impairments, general fatigue, irritability, decreased attention, and decreased productivity. In children, these symptoms have been mistaken for poor motivation or behavior problems. Iron deficiency leads to decreased endurance capacity and submaximal work capacity, including schoolwork, employment, and, yes, athletic performance. It may also have a negative impact on immune function, leading to an increased tendency for infection.

Iron comes in two forms, heme and nonheme. Heme iron, which is found in meat, is much more reliably absorbed than nonheme iron, which is found in plant-based foods. Meat, fish, and poultry contain a factor (MFP factor) that promotes the absorption of nonheme iron from other foods that are eaten at the same time. That's another example of why it's important to eat a variety of foods. Nonheme iron absorption can be further enhanced by eating nonheme-containing foods with foods rich in vitamin C, which can triple the absorption if eaten in the same meal. For example, pair bran flakes, which is a great source of nonheme iron, with an orange, which is a great source of vitamin C. Chili that includes whole tomatoes is another great example. The vitamin C in the tomatoes helps the body absorb the iron in the beans. Think of vitamin C and iron as teammates. They work together to get the job done more efficiently. Table 3.4 is a list of iron-rich foods to work into a meal plan.

A performance meal plan should include enough iron-rich foods to maintain iron stores at an appropriate level to maximize endurance capacity and maintain a healthy immune system.

To review how much iron you need, refer to table 2.4 in chapter 2. Note that vegetarians and youth athletes who avoid animal products may need to increase their overall iron intake to ensure that they are absorbing enough total iron. Vegetarian athletes can calculate the amount of daily iron needed by

Table 3.4 Food Sources of Iron

Food	Serving size	Amount (mg)
Beef, chuck, lean	3 oz	3.2
Chicken, breast, roasted	3 oz	1.1
Turkey, dark meat, roasted	3 oz	2.3
Enriched cereal, 100% iron fortified	3/4 cup	18
Lentils, boiled	1 cup	6.6
Spinach, cooked	1/2 cup	3.2
Black beans, cooked	1/2 cup	1.8
Soybeans, mature, boiled	1/2 cup	4.4
Kidney beans, cooked	1/2 cup	2.6
Oatmeal, instant, fortified	1 cup	10
Raisins, seedless, packed	1/2 cup	1.5
Tofu, raw, firm	1/2 cup	3.4

1 ounce solid = 30 grams; 8 ounces liquid = 240 ml.

multiplying the DRI intake recommendation for their age and sex (see chapter 2) by a factor of 1.8. For example, a 16-year-old female vegetarian dancer needs 15 mg × 1.8 mg/day = 27 mg/day.

Calcium and Vitamin D

Adolescence is a critical time for bone development. Throughout the teenage years, bones are growing longer at a rapid rate as well as gaining density. Calcium is essential for proper bone development, which is why calcium needs are the highest during adolescent years. The more calcium that is deposited in bones during this time, the stronger the bones will be, and strong bones should be a priority for all athletes. Because vitamin D is involved in the absorption and regulation of calcium, both nutrients are critical for bone health. Adolescents who do not get enough calcium or vitamin D compromise the development of peak bone mass, greatly increasing the risk of osteoporosis later in life. Unfortunately, osteoporosis is of little concern to teenagers. As a sport dietitian who specializes in the development of youth athletes, I spend very little time talking about their future health. Instead, I help them understand the importance of strong bones for today and throughout their sport careers. These nutrients help to build a strong skeleton to withstand long hours of practice, training, and competition. This is absolutely necessary for athletes whose bodies take a beating. Injured athletes cannot perform to the best of their abilities. I tell my clients, Take care of your body, and your body will take care of you.

Vitamin D and calcium are well known for their roles in bone health, but both have other important functions in the body. Calcium is important for normal enzyme activity and muscle contraction. The importance of vitamin D in the body has become more evident in recent years. Research suggests that vitamin D has an active role in immune function, protein synthesis, muscle function, inflammatory processes, cell growth, and skeletal muscle regulation. Researchers are busy studying how vitamin D insufficiency and deficiency might negatively affect performance.

Today, it is estimated that over 77 percent of the population is vitamin D insufficient. Although the body can synthesize vitamin D from sunlight, the distance from the equator, season, and time of day make that an unreliable source for some athletes. The production of vitamin D from the sun is also dictated by cloud coverage, pollution, sunblock, skin pigmentation, and age. Mix that with the fact that vitamin D is not found in many foods, and it's clear why deficiency is an issue.

In November 2010, the U.S. Institute of Medicine (IOM) released new recommendations for dietary intake of vitamin D: 400-600 IU per day for children and adults (0-70 years) and 800 IU per day for older adults (>70 years). These values were only slightly increased from previous recommendations, and many experts believe these numbers are still too low. To help meet your calcium and vitamin D needs, pay attention to calcium and vitamin D intake, and eat a variety of foods that offer these nutrients. In addition, consider having your vitamin D level checked at your next routine physical examination. If you have a low vitamin D level, dietary supplementation may be necessary, but it should be done under the supervision of a physician or registered dietitian. Table 3.5 lists the amount of calcium in average portion sizes of common calcium-rich foods, and table 3.6 lists food sources of vitamin D. To review how much calcium and vitamin D youth need, refer to the table 2.4 in chapter 2.

Table 3.5   Food Sources of Calcium

Food	Serving size	Amount (mg)
Cow's milk	1 cup	300
Yogurt, Greek, nonfat	5.2 oz	160
Broccoli, chopped	1 cup	62
Orange juice, calcium fortified*	4 oz	~175
Cheddar cheese	1 oz	204
Frozen waffle, whole grain	1	196
Tofu	1/2 cup	275
Kale, cooked	1/2 cup	90
Soybeans, mature, cooked	1/2 cup	88
White beans, canned, cooked	1/2 cup	96

*Check label; amounts vary by brand.

*1 ounce solid = 30 grams; 8 ounces liquid = 240 ml.

Table 3.6 Food Sources of Vitamin D

Food	Serving size	Amount (in IU)
Swordfish	3 oz	566
Salmon, sockeye, cooked	3 oz	447
Tuna, canned, in water	3 oz	154
Orange juice, vitamin D fortified*	~1 cup	137
Cow's milk, vitamin D fortified	1 cup	115-124
Yogurt, vitamin D fortified	6 oz	~80 (varies)
Margarine, vitamin D fortified	~ 1 tbsp	60
Sardines, canned in oil, drained	2 sardines	46
Liver, beef, cooked	3 oz	42
Egg	1 large (vitamin D is in the yolk)	41
Dry cereal, vitamin D fortified	~ 3/4 cup	~40 (amounts vary per brand and variety)
Swiss cheese	1 oz	6

*Check label; amounts vary by brand.

*1 ounce solid = 30 grams; 8 ounces liquid = 240 ml.

Hydration for Active Youth

If there is a section of this book to read and read again, this is it. The fluid intake and hydration status of a youth athlete are critical and not to be taken lightly. There is no cheaper, simpler, or more effective way to help performance and protect health than staying hydrated during exercise.

As you learned in chapter 2, water is the most vital nutrient and plays a key role in maintaining health and performance. In adults, a loss of 2 percent body weight in fluids has been shown to have adverse effects on performance. In children, those negative effects are thought to occur sooner, with just a 1 percent decrease in body weight. This is especially true when exercising in hot and humid conditions. The effects associated with dehydration in children lead to decreased endurance and performance by negatively affecting the cardiovascular system, thermoregulation, and central fatigue or perceived exhaustion. Dehydration is dangerous, and it can be deadly.

The goal of hydration is the same for all youth athletes: to prevent dehydration and optimize performance. This can be a hard sell for athletes who need to make weight, but it really should not be. Maintaining a healthy hydration status is the first priority in any performance plan.

Fluid Needs for Youth Athletes

As with nutrients, the DRIs give us an idea of how much water is needed daily. The RDA is for *total* water; that is, what we take in from foods, beverages, and drinking water. Youth athletes need to consume more fluids to support their increased activity. In an ideal world, athletes would be able to drink enough fluid during activity to keep pace with their sweat rates. Unfortunately, that's not always possible. First, not all athletes know their sweat rates. Second, athletes who sweat heavily cannot realistically drink enough fluid while exercising to maintain a balance. The fastest way for athletes to learn how much fluid they need to drink after exercise is to weigh themselves before and after training sessions. Knowing how much fluid is lost during activity will help them individualize their hydration plans. To determine fluid loss, use this simple formula:

1. Weigh yourself nude immediately before exercise.
2. Weight: _____
3. Track your fluid consumed during exercise.
4. Fluid consumption: _____
5. Weigh yourself nude immediately after exercise.
6. Weight: _____
7. Subtract your weight after exercise from your weight before exercise to determine the number of pounds lost.
8. Pounds lost: _____
9. Multiply the number of pounds lost by 3 to determine the number of cups of fluid to drink after exercise.
10. Cups of fluid to drink: _____

Or if using kilograms, subtract weight after from the weight before to determine the kg lost. For every 2.2 kg lost, drink 720 ml of fluid.

In addition to calculating fluid losses during activity, youth athletes should be familiar with evaluating their urine color. A urine chart is a simple tool for assessing whether you are drinking enough to stay hydrated. As a general rule, pale yellow urine (like lemonade) indicates being fairly well hydrated, whereas darker yellow urine (like apple juice) indicates potential dehydration. Coaches, trainers, and athletes should have a urine chart visible. I advise coaches and trainers to have a poster hanging in workout areas and athletes to consider purchasing a pocket guide. (They are available for purchase at www.hydrationcheck.com.)

It's also important for youth athletes to know the signs and symptoms of dehydration. They can be vague, but athletes who know what to look for will be able to identify them. Warning signs and symptoms of dehydration include headache and light-headedness, noticeable thirst, irritability, nausea, muscle cramping, dark yellow urine, difficulty paying attention, and weakness and fatigue resulting in decreased performance.

Hydration Guidelines for Youth Athletes

As with nutrient recommendations, adequate water intakes for athletes are much more researched in adults than in children and adolescents. The most recent hydration recommendations from the American Academy of Pediatrics (Council on Sports Medicine and Fitness and Council on School Health et al., 2011) are as follows:

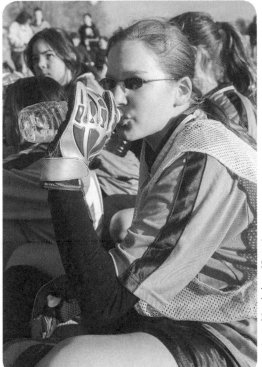

There is no cheaper, simpler, or more effective way to help performance and protect your health than staying hydrated during exercise.

Nancy Louie/iStockphoto/Getty Images

- Provide and promote the consumption of readily accessible fluids at regular intervals before, during, and after activity to offset sweat losses and maintain adequate hydration while avoiding overdrinking.

- Encourage children to drink during activity. Generally that means 100 to 250 milliliters (3-8 ounces) every 20 minutes for 9- to 12-year-olds and up to 1.5 liters (34-50 ounces) per hour for adolescent athletes to minimize sweat-induced body-water deficits during exercise as long as preactivity hydration status is good.

- Consider weighing before and after activity to assess fluid losses. Pre- and postactivity body-weight measurements can help you understand how much fluid is being lost during activity so that you have more information for individual rehydration needs.

- Electrolyte-supplemented beverages that emphasize sodium may be warranted during long-duration (≥1 hour), repeated same-day sessions of strenuous exercise, sports participation, and hot weather.

- Educate children and adolescents on the merits of ample hydration.

- Youth sport governing bodies, tournament directors, and other event administrators should provide adequate rest and recovery periods of two or more hours between same-day contests in warm to hot weather to allow sufficient recovery and rehydration.

Adapted from American Academy of Pediatrics Council on Sports Medicine and Fitness and Council on School Health, 2011, "Policy statement—Climatic heat stress and exercising children and adolescents," *Pediatrics* 128(3): e741-e747.

Fuel Focus

Mary

Mary, a 15-year-old competitive cheerleader, came to see me with complaints of fatigue and headaches during practice. Mary's mom was concerned because Mary was having trouble getting through practice without feeling ill. The more I listened to Mary, the more concerned I was about her fluid status. All of her symptoms pointed to dehydration.

Mary explained that she drinks very little. As she explained it, she and her teammates were permitted water breaks only when they performed their routines perfectly. Apparently, water was the team's reward for getting it right. Mary's mom was right to be concerned.

Mary's cheerleading coach may have thought that he was teaching the team a lesson, but instead he was creating a dangerous environment. Keeping fluids from athletes, especially youth athletes, when performance is poor is abusive. Mary's mom admitted that she thought it was too tough, but she didn't want to step on the coach's toes. I advised Mary's mom to talk to the coach about the hydration plan we created. I also encouraged her to invite him to call me with any questions or concerns. Simply discussing this with the coach resolved the problem. By speaking up, Mary's mom helped other youth athletes on the team who may have been less likely to do so.

Notice the recommendation to educate children and adolescents on the importance of getting adequate hydration. Coaches, trainers, and parents have the role of helping youth athletes understand why hydration is important. But telling them they need to drink is not enough. A study by Cleary and colleagues (2012) assessed the hydration status and behaviors of adolescent athletes both before and after a one-time educational intervention, then compared it to a prescribed hydration intervention. It showed that the single education session did not result in hydration behavior changes, but prescribing individualized hydration protocols did. This study supports the need to go above and beyond simply telling young athletes to drink more; they need to be shown exactly how to do it.

Before we conclude this section, note the following situations and conditions in which fluid requirements are higher and require additional attention:

- Competing in extreme weather conditions, wearing heavy equipment, or competing at altitude
- Being ill or having been ill recently, especially if it involves gastrointestinal (GI) distress (vomiting, diarrhea), fever, or both
- Taking medications that may contribute to decreased exercise tolerance
- Having known medical conditions

Both hot and humid weather and cold weather pose a significant risk for dehydration. Although it may seem counterintuitive, exercising outside in the cold can put athletes at even greater risk for dehydration than exercising in the heat. Being bundled up or covered in heavy equipment makes it harder to gauge fluid loss than when sweat is visibly collecting on skin or clothes. Exercise performed in the heat can result in measurable dehydration if sweat losses are not adequately replaced. For the safety of all youth athletes, parents, coaches, and trainers should have water or other appropriate fluids readily accessible, and youth athletes should be given regular opportunities throughout athletic activities to hydrate and offset sweat losses.

Creating a Hydration Schedule

Even with the best intentions, staying hydrated during activity can be a challenge. Setting up a daily hydration schedule can help youth athletes get in the habit of drinking fluids at regular times throughout the day. Athletes should start with a basic fluid schedule, as shown in table 3.7, and then tailor it to their individual activity levels and hydration needs.

Table 3.7 Hydration Schedule

Time of day	Fluid intake
Upon waking through bedtime	Fill your water bottle. Drink 8 oz of water first thing in the morning, and aim for 6 to 8 oz every hour after.
2 hours before exercise	Drink at least 2 cups (16 oz) in this hour. Drinking 2 to 3 hours before exercise allows enough time for fluid to be lost through urine before exercise begins.
30 minutes before exercise	Drink 5 to 10 oz of fluid. There is no benefit to chugging fluid in an attempt to stay hydrated. Although people differ, the body can absorb fluid only so fast, and you do not want to have extra fluid sloshing around in your stomach when it is time to start your activity.
Immediately before exercise	Check your weight.
Every 15 minutes during exercise	*Keep track of how much total fluid you consumed. It can be helpful to start with a full water bottle so you can quickly assess how much you drank. *Drink 4 to 8 oz every 15 minutes, or 16 to 32 oz over an hour, without overloading the body and causing GI distress. Remember, one gulp is about 1 oz, so aim for 4 to 8 gulps of fluid every 15 minutes.
After exercise	Reweigh yourself immediately after exercise. Compare that weight to your preactivity weight to see how much water you lost.

8 ounces liquid = 240 ml.

Water Versus Sport Drink: Which Do Athletes Need?

As athletes perspire, they lose electrolytes, especially sodium and chloride, the two minerals found in the greatest concentrations in sweat. Along with water, these electrolytes need to be replaced to prevent fluid imbalance. Sodium is the electrolyte of biggest concern. It is needed to maintain fluid balance and prevent cramping. Sodium enhances fluid retention, so it helps to maintain hydration. It also stimulates thirst. Water alone will not replace electrolytes. As a general rule, athletes who participate in continuous activity for more than one hour may benefit from more than water.

If an athlete prefers to drink water, find out why. By asking questions, I have learned a lot about why youth athletes drink plain water. Sometimes it has nothing to do with nutrition. For example, a 17-year-old female hockey goalie came to see me to improve her sport nutrition plan before heading off to college. Although she was on the ice for the entire game and would have benefited from a sport drink, she reported that she drank only water during games. When I asked why, she said that she did not want to stain her uniform. She had only seconds between plays to squirt fluid into her mouth through her mask; if she missed, red or bright orange sport drink covered her white uniform. I suggested a homemade colorless sport drink. Problem solved.

Another young athlete, a 14-year-old high school wrestler, filled his water bottle only with water for a different reason. Although he sweated heavily and his weekly practices lasted over two hours, his high school wrestling coach did not allow sport drink. He was concerned that the athletes would spill them, causing the mats to get sticky. Although it was a viable concern, we needed a solution that would help this wrestler get the fluid, electrolyte, and carbohydrate replacement he needed to train properly during practice. I suggested to the coach to have the athletes fill their water bottles with sport drink, and then keep them in a designated area away from the mats. Luckily, the coach was on board with good nutrition and agreed to come up with a plan.

Research has shown that when children and adolescents are given only water to drink, they do not replace their fluid losses as completely as when they are offered flavored drinks or sport drinks. Youth athletes who struggle to drink enough can benefit from sport drinks. The sodium in sport drinks not only replaces sodium losses but also heightens the desire to drink more, resulting in better overall hydration. Some athletes sweat heavily and may require more sodium to replace their losses. Following are signs of being a heavy sweater:

- Stinging eyes when sweat drips into them
- Salty-tasting sweat
- Feeling gritty after a long bout of exercise or a long run
- White streaks on face, arms, and upper back after exercise

Sport drinks are not the only way to replace electrolytes. Eating the right foods before, during, and after activity can also replace electrolytes. Chapter 5 discusses the specifics of fueling and hydrating for game day, including how to increase sodium intake through foods.

If used properly, sport drinks can be very beneficial for youth athletes. Their purpose is to provide fluid, carbohydrate, and electrolytes during and after sport activity. Drinking them for breakfast or while watching television only adds calories and sodium that may not be needed. Water is the best beverage for other times of the day.

As mentioned at the beginning of the chapter, before developing a sport nutrition plan for a youth athlete, it is important to clearly identify the goal. Yes, added protein is needed to build muscle, but simply pounding protein will not build muscle. Likewise, an athlete looking to reduce body fat should not simply eat less. Doing so could result in decreased athletic performance and may lead to nutrient deficiencies. There is a right way and a wrong way to do everything. Chapter 4 provides tips and tricks for altering body composition in a safe, healthy, and achievable way.

Adjusting Body Composition to Reach Your Goals

Many athletes attempt to gain a competitive edge by changing their body composition. And it makes sense. When it comes to athletic performance, there are benefits and drawbacks to being a certain size. Take height, for example. Taller people tend to be more successful in basketball, a sport in which reaching a level high above the floor is required. Shorter people tend to have an advantage in sports such as gymnastics, in which a lower center of gravity can promote better balance. Body weight, as well as the ratio of body fat to lean muscle mass, also influences performance. Excessive body fat can be a disadvantage because it adds to the load carried by the body. In contrast, very low body fat levels can have negative effects not only on sport performance but also on overall health.

As with many things in life, there is a right way and a wrong way to alter body composition. If you do it right, you will feel better, look better, and perform better. If you do it wrong, you might look better or be satisfied with the number on the scale, but the results will likely be short-lived, and your health and social well-being may suffer. Body composition alterations should be undertaken to improve sport performance, not for other reasons that may compromise health or well-being.

Weight Gain and Muscular Development the Right Way

For many young athletes, especially those in sports in which size dominates, weight gain cannot come fast enough. Athletes in these sports gain an advantage from the increased power and strength that increased body mass can

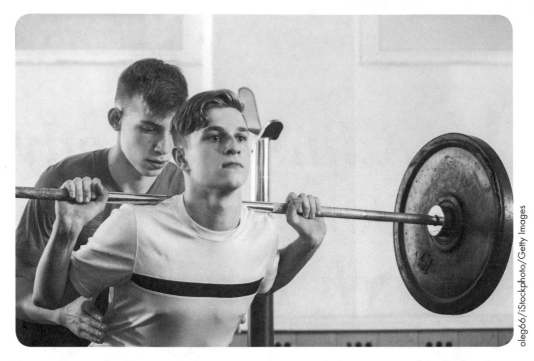

oleg66/iStockphoto/Getty Images

Training the muscles from a young age can improve strength, but it is not until the body is developmentally mature enough that weight gain from lean body mass should be the primary goal.

provide. Although obesity is a big issue in the younger generation today, many youth athletes struggle to gain weight; when they do gain, it can be a challenge to keep it on.

Aside from the normal weight gain that occurs as adolescents age, weight gain can occur as the result of increased fat, increased muscle, or both. Even the youngest of athletes can gain body fat by eating enough calories; gaining muscle mass is a different story and a bigger challenge. As you learned in chapter 1, teenagers develop at different rates. Although training your muscles from a young age can result in improved strength, only when the body is developmentally ready should real muscle growth be the focus. Once the body is mature enough and levels of testosterone peak in males, the training regimen and eating plan can be adapted to focus on building muscle mass and bulking up.

Determining Objectives for Weight Gain

Gaining weight requires taking in enough calories for growth, development, and activity and then eating more. Some youth athletes consume a lot of additional calories. But as mentioned earlier, the eating plan should support the training plan. Muscles do not develop by simply eating more calories or protein. To increase mass, muscles must be worked, and the harder they work, the more calories they need. Determining exactly how many calories to consume can be tricky. Genetics, body type, and metabolic rate all play a role in how many calories are burned, and the goal of the athlete must be considered. Some athletes want only to increase muscle mass, whereas others may need to build muscle mass as well as slightly increase body fat. Let's take a closer look at both of these goals.

Increasing Muscle Mass Only

Mark, a 17-year-old sprinter, was referred to me by his track and field coach. Mark had a short stature and lean build and was looking to increase his muscle mass to be more powerful. He had a great strength and conditioning program in place but did not have a nutrition plan that properly supported his training. Like many youth athletes, Mark didn't think too much about what he ate. He ate when he was hungry and didn't eat when he wasn't. Mark needed a balanced nutrition plan that provided enough energy to support his training while balancing and timing his protein intake to maximize muscle growth. Here's what we came up with:

Goal: Increase skeletal mass.

Why: Increase strength and power output.

How: Develop a meal plan that optimizes when and how much carbohydrate he eats, especially around training; spread protein intake evenly for each meal and mini-meal throughout the entire day; monitor body fat and body weight to make sure he is gaining muscle and not body fat.

Increasing Muscle Mass and Body Fat

Jack, a 6-foot 3-inch (190 cm) 17-year-old junior hockey player, came to see me for weight gain. His personal goal was to gain 20 pounds (9 kg) before his next season so he would be bigger, stronger, and more competitive on the ice. His weight was 178 pounds (81 kg). Like many competitive athletes of his size, he complained of losing weight at the beginning of each season. He had some classic symptoms of adolescent athletes who struggle to gain weight: He would eat large amounts of food at some meals but forget to eat at other times of the day. Although he could eat a lot, if he didn't feel hungry, he didn't think about food.

Jack needed a plan for eating enough to support his offseason training, which included four days of heavy lifting and other cross-training, but less cardiorespiratory activity than normal. He needed a meal plan that showed him not only how much food he needed to eat but also how to balance the macronutrients so that he would eat enough at each meal and still feel hungry three or four hours later. Jack also needed tips on increasing his caloric intake to support growth and muscular development, not just gain body fat. I set him up on a plan that provided enough calories to support his growth, development, and energy expenditure as well as the extra calories to build new muscle tissue. Because Jack's energy expenditure increases so drastically once his hockey season starts, we discussed how to eat enough calories for muscular development as well as slightly increase his body fat percentage in anticipation of the start of his season. We also discussed how to adjust his meal plan during the season so that he could maintain his gains. Here's what we came up with:

Goal: Increase skeletal mass and slightly increase body fat.

Why: Increase overall size and strength so that he would be more competitive on the ice; anticipate a decrease in body fat once his season starts.

How: Develop a meal plan showing Jack how to eat enough of the right foods at the right times to support his normal growth and development as well as his training; teach him how to prevent weight loss once his season starts.

Tracking Calories to Monitor Weight Gain

So how do you go about eating enough of the right foods to support your increased training load? For starters, you need to have a plan that shows how much food you need. If you recall from chapter 3, table 3.1 provides the estimated energy requirements (EER) for females and males ages 8 to 18. Remember that estimated energy requirement (EER) is based on energy expenditure, requirements for growth, and level of physical activity. If the goal is weight gain, you may need more. I have worked with young athletes who needed anywhere from 2,000 to 5,500 calories per day to reach their body composition and performance goals. That's a huge range. To prevent overeating, you'll need to do some homework. Follow these steps to create a plan for yourself:

1. Track Your Weight

First, you need to be very clear about what is happening with your weight. Remember that as a growing adolescent, you should be gaining some weight to account for basic growth and development. The weight you want to gain is in addition to that.

2. Determine Your Current Intake

Next, keep a food journal of everything you eat and drink for four or five days. An easy way is to get a notebook and write down the fluids and foods you take in. You can download or use online a variety of apps to track intake. Table 4.1 shows the information to include in a food journal. Once you have four or five days' worth of data, you are ready to calculate your current caloric intake. How you adjust your caloric intake will depend on your recent weight history.

- If you have been losing weight, you need more calories. First, compare your current intake to that on the EER table in chapter 3. If you are not eating what is recommended on the EER table, start by increasing your caloric intake to that amount. Follow that for two weeks and see if you continue to lose weight. If you are still losing weight, increase your calories by 500 per day.

- If you have been maintaining your weight, you need more calories. Average your current intake over the past four or five days and add 500 calories per day. Track your intake and weight over the next two weeks. Your progress will determine whether to repeat step 1, move to step 3, or maintain this amount as your new daily caloric intake.

- If you have been gaining weight, but not fast enough, you need more calories. Average your current intake over the past four or five days and take in an additional 300 to 400 calories per day. Track your intake and weight over the next two weeks. If this increase in calories does not result in a proper weight gain, add 300 more calories per day and repeat this step.

3. Track Your Body Fat

Finally, remember that just because the number on the scale is going up does not mean that you are gaining muscle mass. It is important to track your body fat percentage to make sure you are progressing toward your goal. If you are trying to increase skeletal muscle mass and body fat, you should see both the

Table 4.1 Food Journal Daily Entry

Time of day	Food	Fluid	Comments
6:00 a.m.	1 cup oatmeal with 1 tsp cinnamon, 1 tbsp raisins, 1 cup 2% milk	8 oz orange juice	
9:00 a.m.	1 green apple (medium size) with 2 tbsp peanut butter	Two 24 oz bottles of water	
12:00 p.m.	1 grilled chicken breast salad: 4 oz grilled chicken 3 cups romaine 2 tomatoes 2 tbsp parmesan cheese 2 tbsp sunflower seeds 2 tbsp vinaigrette dressing	8 oz water 12 oz chocolate milk	Homemade chocolate milk with 3 tbsp syrup
3:00 p.m.	2 slices turkey breast, 2 slices whole-wheat bread, 2 tbsp mayo, 1 oz Swiss cheese		Costco brand bread
6:00 p.m.	5 oz hamburger on wheat bun with lettuce, tomato, ketchup, mustard 16 grapes 1 baked potato with 2 tbsp margarine	24 oz water	Hamburger was at Friday's restaurant
9:00 p.m.	17 pretzel sticks	12 oz apple juice	Salted pretzels

1 ounce solid = 30 grams; 8 ounces liquid = 240 ml.

number on the scale and your body fat percentage going up. If your goal is to increase only skeletal muscle mass, tracking body fat is an even bigger priority. In both cases, you should be noticing body composition changes as well as strength improvements.

Body fat percentage can be measured by a variety of methods. Bioelectrical impedance is a simple and cost-effective way to monitor body fat at home. A skinfold measurement can be done as well, but it should be done by a trained administrator. More sophisticated equipment, such as underwater weighing in a hydrostatic tank or a Bod Pod, is often available only in academic or clinical settings.

Employing Strategies for Weight Gain

Determining the amount of food you need to eat is not easy, but once you figure it out, you have another challenge: figuring out how to eat all of that food. I've worked with some male athletes who needed over 5,000 calories per day. Eating all of those calories at the right time and with the right combination of nutrients can be a challenge, especially when you have to plan your eating around school, practice, sporting events, and sleep. Weight-gain success requires planning, preparation, and a commitment to your goals. The sections that follow offer some strategies for eating more without feeling like you just ate Thanksgiving dinner every day. Also, part IV of this book provides some recipes for high-calorie energy bars, snacks, and smoothies to help you reach your goals.

Eat More Meals, More Often

Divide your calories into six or seven meals and mini-meals throughout the day. Forget breakfast, lunch, and dinner. Youth athletes who struggle to gain weight need many meals, starting first thing in the morning and continuing until it's time to go to bed. When I plan meals for athletes, I refer to meal 1, meal 2, meal 3, meal 4, meal 5, and meal 6, and then I add preworkout, workout, and postworkout calories, if necessary. Because building muscle is the goal, include 20 to 30 grams of protein at each meal. (Females and those with lower calorie requirements should be on the lower end, and males and those with higher calorie requirements should be on the higher end.)

Increase Portion Sizes

It is possible to increase your food intake by 500 calories per day simply by eating five or so bites more of the foods you already eat. If you are eating the right foods already, this can be an easy way to add calories.

Add Liquid Calories

Liquids move through the stomach faster than solid foods and therefore don't have the same satiety factor. Although you may not think of it this way, a 600- to 700-calorie smoothie counts as one of your meals.

Drink Beverages Other Than Water

This will not count as a meal, but drinking a sport drink during activity can be an effective way to add a few hundred calories without thinking too much about it. If you are trying to gain muscle, even shorter training sessions can use the support of extra carbohydrate.

Add Extras

Adding toppers to foods that you already eat is an easy way to boost calories. Here are some suggestions:

- Add nuts, seeds, and dried fruits to morning oatmeal, yogurt, salads, or smoothies.
- Add a tablespoon of olive oil and honey to your smoothie or oatmeal.
- Add nut butter, hummus, avocado, or pesto to crackers or sandwiches.
- Add shredded or grated cheese to potatoes, salads, soups, pasta dishes, and vegetables.

Eating enough calories is critical for weight gain, but eating the right balance of nutrients can make reaching your goal a lot easier. Loading up on pizza, fries, and wings might seem like a simple solution to gaining weight, but those foods won't necessarily help you gain the lean muscle mass you are looking for. Foods high in dietary fat can fill you up fast and leave you feeling full for hours after eating. That's not an ideal situation for an athlete who needs to eat often. The same is true of consuming too much protein. Protein increases satiety, so consuming too much can displace other nutrients, such as the carbohydrate that working muscles need. Recall from chapter 3 that each nutrient has a place in the meal plan, which should be balanced according to your goals.

Decreasing Body Fat Without Dieting

Because coaches, trainers, and parents play an important role in helping youth athletes be the best they can be at their sports, they need to be careful when communicating body composition goals. This is especially true in the case of athletes who may benefit from decreasing body fat. Youth athletes often feel pressured to lose weight to perform better or look better. If not communicated properly, the suggestion to lose weight can crush an athlete's confidence and lead to negative feelings and harmful eating behaviors.

At a recent Eating Disorders in Sports Conference, the speakers included a variety of former athletes who had suffered from eating disorders that destroyed their careers. Many of them reported that their decision to lose weight was triggered by a remark made by a parent, coach, or teammate about how they could perform better if they weighed less. Although these remarks were likely well intentioned, they led to unfortunate consequences for these athletes who wanted to succeed.

As you learned in chapter 1, the body goes through tremendous changes during puberty, and not all of those changes can be controlled. Female athletes especially may be uncomfortable with the additional body fat that accompanies puberty. They need reassurance that this is normal. Body composition is not only a reflection of eating habits; it is partially controlled by genetics. Not all athletes will be able to achieve the physiques they want without sacrificing their health, which in turn sacrifices performance. Too much focus on weight loss can be devastating to preadolescent athletes' self-esteem and confidence. Instead, a plan should be put in place that shows them how to eat the right foods for health and performance while allowing height to catch up to weight. For older adolescent athletes who can really benefit from a reduction in body fat, a plan that sets realistic and achievable goals can result in big benefits.

Determining Weight-Loss Objectives

Losing body fat requires creating an energy deficit. Because caloric intake also influences athletic performance, growth, development, and mood, a weight-loss plan requires serious consideration. Dieting is discouraged; rather, a healthy eating plan targeted at supporting performance is highly encouraged. Some athletes may wish only to decrease body fat; others may wish to decrease body fat while increasing skeletal muscle mass. Let's take a closer look at both of these goals.

Decreasing Body Fat Only

Amber, a 15-year-old lacrosse player, came to see me for weight loss. She was a fantastic player with incredible strength, but her weight was slowing her down and limiting her endurance. Amber was a classic endomorph body type with a heavy bone structure and a propensity for gaining weight. To her benefit, she also built muscle easily. Still, she was 5 feet 2 inches (157 cm) and 135 pounds (61 kg), and I agreed that we could improve her speed on the field if we made a few tweaks to her meal plan to promote a small, steady weight loss that did not disrupt her performance. She practiced six days a week for two hours a day. Amber also told me that she was hungry all the time. Her mom was very involved and supportive and was trying her best to give her an adequate diet. She had read online that chocolate milk was good for recovery, so she would make sure that Amber had a 20-ounce (600 ml) bottle after every workout. Amber's mom also made sure she was well stocked with sport drinks throughout the day and always carried snacks to have between meals.

It was clear that Amber's diet had a lot of room for improvement. She was drinking a lot of fluids that provided a lot of low-nutrient calories. I suspected that Amber was hungry so often because of her high intake of simple-sugar liquid calories. She needed a meal plan that provided more lean protein and more fiber to help her feel full. By rearranging her meals and balancing her nutrition, she would feel more satiated with fewer calories. Not only would she lose weight, but she would also feel and perform better. Amber learned a lot in our time working together. We created meal plans she could follow that met her needs and helped fuel her sport performance. The result of following the meal plan was a small, steady weight loss and improved energy and speed. Here's what we came up with:

Goal: Decrease body fat.

Why: Improve speed.

How: Create a meal plan that shows Amber how to balance nutrition properly over the course of the day using foods that would not only nourish her body but also help her feel full. Cut out a lot, but not all, of the simple sugar in her diet. After she learned about the purpose of sport drinks, she realized that drinking them in school was not beneficial, but having one during practice was.

Decreasing Body Fat and Increasing Skeletal Muscle Mass

Jill, a 16-year-old rower, came to see me because she wanted to lose weight and build muscle. Jill was not referred to me by her coach, but she told me that being bigger than the other girls made her feel uncomfortable. She believed that she could contribute more to the team if she weighed less and was stronger. Jill was a positive, knowledgeable young athlete and had a great body image. I agreed that a slight reduction in body fat would result in a noticeable benefit, and she did not have far to go. Slightly decreasing her body fat percentage while providing adequate nutrition to build muscle would increase her strength and power and give her a performance benefit. As a rower, she needed carbohydrate to fuel her performance. We would need to create an energy deficit to promote weight loss while providing the right nutrients to build or maintain her current muscle mass. That meant a plan with more protein, but we had to make sure we did not exceed her total caloric intake, and fat would need to be low. The plan would provide adequate energy for growth, development, and energy expenditure while creating a small deficit to promote fat loss.

Jill understood the fine line between decreasing body fat and improving muscle mass. She was committed to the plan and understood that the number on the scale would be slow to change. She agreed to use her mirror and performance rather than her scale to monitor her progress. She focused on meal balance and timing and made sure she fueled by day and around activity and decreased her intake later in the day. I monitored her body fat using a simple body fat monitor. Within three months, Jill was at her goal.

Goal: Decrease body fat.

Why: Feel better about her appearance, increase rowing power.

How: Follow a meal plan that provides enough carbohydrate to fuel her higher-intensity training, limit fat to allow for a proper caloric deficit without limiting the fuel needed for performance, and have protein at every meal to ensure adequate intake for building lean skeletal mass and increasing mealtime satiety.

Discussing Weight Loss the Right Way

What is the right way to discuss body composition concerns with a youth athlete? First, it's important to determine whether weight loss is appropriate. Remember from chapter 1 that the body undergoes significant changes in weight and body fat composition before and during puberty. These changes are normal and necessary for healthy growth and development. Parents, coaches, and trainers may not be the best people to evaluate whether a young athlete's weight is appropriate. Instead, this topic can be taken up with a pediatrician during an annual physical exam or sport participation exam.

There is not one perfect way to determine healthy weight ranges, but tools are available. Body mass index (BMI), a common and practical method, can be calculated for children, teens, and adults, although it is used slightly differently for children and teens. For children and teens, BMI is used to screen for potential weight- and health-related issues and is shown as percentages plotted on growth charts, relative to others of the same sex and age. The drastic body composition changes that occur at various ages and stages make using only this tool problematic for determining a true weight problem. Remember that both males and females show normal increases in body fat in preparation for puberty. Because BMI does not account for lean muscle mass, a child or teen can have a high BMI for his age and sex but not have a weight problem. For example, a 16-year-old male with considerable muscle mass and low body fatness may have a high weight and therefore a higher BMI than other males his age with lower muscle mass. Nevertheless, BMI is easy to determine and is a starting point for assessing body weight appropriateness. If BMI is high, other tools can be used to assess body fatness. A health care practitioner can give further guidance.

To find a youth athlete's BMI, obtain an accurate height and weight and plot it on the growth chart for boys (see figure 4.1a) or girls (see figure 4.1b).

Tracking Calories to Monitor Weight Loss

Once you have determined that weight loss is appropriate, it is time to determine the goal as it relates to athletic performance. Should fat loss be the only focus, or would gaining muscle mass improve performance? Are you developmentally ready to focus on building mass? As mentioned, dieting is discouraged. All attention should be on building a healthy eating plan that will result in a performance benefit. As with trying to gain weight, it is important to do a little homework to ensure a proper plan. How you adjust your caloric intake will depend on your recent weight history and eating patterns. Follow these steps:

1. Track Your Weight

First, you need to be very clear about what is happening with your weight. Remember that as a growing adolescent, you should be gaining some weight

2 to 20 years: Boys
Body mass index-for-age percentiles

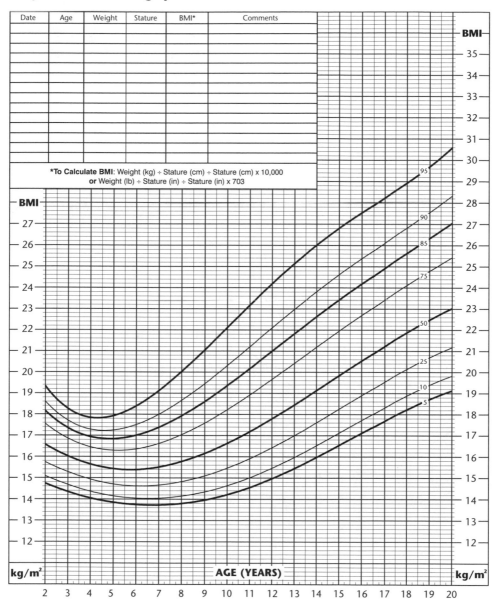

Figure 4.1a Body mass index-for-age chart for boys.
Source: Developed by the National Center for Health Statistics in collaboration with the National Center for Chronic Disease Prevention and Health Promotion (2000). http://www.cdc.gov/growthcharts
From H.R. Mangieri, 2017, *Fueling young athletes* (Champaign, IL: Human Kinetics).

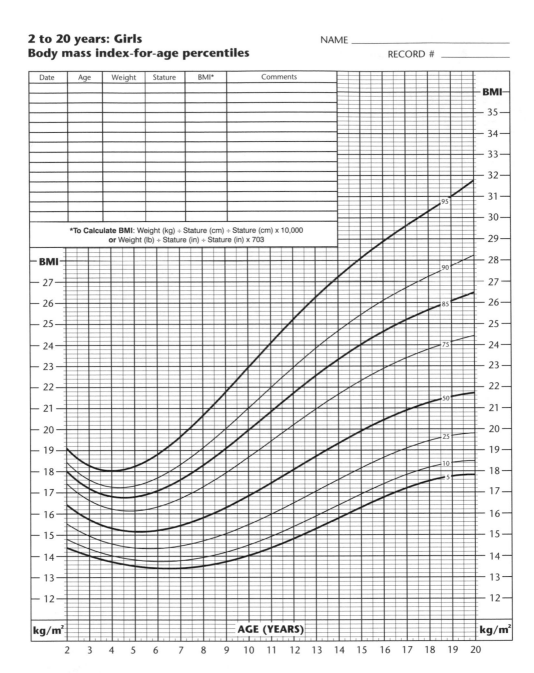

Figure 4.1*b* Body mass index-for-age chart for girls.
Source: Developed by the National Center for Health Statistics in collaboration with the National Center for Chronic Disease Prevention and Health Promotion (2000). http://www.cdc.gov/growthcharts
From H.R. Mangieri, 2017, *Fueling young athletes* (Champaign, IL: Human Kinetics).

to account for basic growth and development. Depending on your height and stage of development, an appropriate goal might be to maintain your weight and allow your height to catch up.

2. Determine Your Current Intake

Next, keep a food journal of everything you eat and drink for four or five days (see table 4.1 for a sample daily entry in a food journal). You can use this information to calculate your current caloric intake as well as to identify trends in your eating. Putting a performance plan together to meet your body composition goals is not only about eating less; it is also about rearranging your current meals and snacks so that you get the most out of your calories.

- If you have been gaining weight, you probably need fewer calories. First, compare your current intake to that on the EER table 3.1. If you are eating more than what is recommended on the EER table, start by decreasing your caloric intake to that amount. Follow that for two weeks and see if you continue to gain weight. If you are still gaining weight, a further caloric deficit may be needed. Remember, these calories will not be reduced by dieting; they will be reduced using the strategies discussed in the next section. The caloric deficit that is created will vary based on how many calories over the recommended amount you are eating. Every athlete needs enough calories for adequate growth and development and should never reduce below the recommended calorie guidelines.

- If you have been maintaining your weight but need to lose, depending on your developmental age, focusing on continual weight maintenance is an appropriate approach to changing body composition. Remember that weight gain during the adolescent years is normal and healthy. As you grow taller, your body composition changes; many athletes slim down naturally. If weight loss is necessary, a small reduction in calories (e.g., 200 to 300 per day) may be enough to promote a slow, steady weight loss without negative performance consequences. Track your intake and weight over the next two weeks. Your progress will determine whether you need to repeat step 2, move to step 3, or maintain this amount as your new daily caloric intake.

- If you have been losing weight, but not fast enough for you, maintain your current intake, but continue to track with a food journal. Compare the number of calories you consume with the estimated energy requirements (EER) in table 3.1. There is not a standard for how much weight should be lost in a week. One pound (0.5 kg) per week is an appropriate goal for reducing body fat. If your goal is to reduce body fat but gain muscle, you need to do more than just monitor body weight.

3. Track Your Body Fat

Finally, remember that just because the number on the scale is going down does not mean that you are losing fat mass. When possible and age appropriate, track your body fat percentage to make sure you are progressing toward your goal. If you are trying to increase skeletal muscle mass and decrease body fat, you should see your body fat go down, but the number on the scale might not change. If your goal is only to decrease body fat, both body fat and body weight should decrease. In both cases, you should be noticing body composition changes and performance improvements, and you should have more energy.

Employing Strategies for Weight Loss

Youth athletes are unique. They require all of the nutrition of other growing adolescents, plus more. If nutrient deficiencies occur, their symptoms can appear more dramatic, because they negatively affect performance. This is all the more reason to avoid dieting or any quick-fix weight-loss strategies. Instead, youth athletes should focus on modifying how and what they eat. With each new week in my practice, I see the negative consequences dieting can cause: negative feelings toward food and body image, disordered eating, weight loss that becomes out of control, fatigue, fractures and bone injuries, gastrointestinal issues, and lifelong struggles with weight obsession and yo-yo dieting. More and more young female athletes are choosing to go gluten free or vegan but without guidance. It is dangerous to eliminate food groups without replacing the nutrients the eliminated foods contain.

Fuel Focus

Tim

Tim, a 16-year-old baseball player, had just started his season and was not performing as well as he had last year. His hitting was strong, but he was struggling to get to the bases fast enough. He had spent his time between competition seasons focusing on building muscle but did not do much cardiorespiratory training. He gained weight in the form of both muscle and body fat, resulting in improved strength and decreased speed. His strength and conditioning coach referred him to me for weight-loss help.

When Tim came to see me, he was overweight. I agreed that he would benefit from reducing his body fat; however, doing so in the middle of his busy season, when the focus should be eating for performance, would be a challenge. I worked with Tim to create a performance plan but advised him to set up an appointment with me during the transition period of his training year, when his preparation and competition were over.

Taking in fewer calories than are expended is critical for weight loss, but the body still needs to meet the daily recommended intakes to prevent deficiencies and negative performance effects. As calories are reduced, you can begin to feel hunger that you have not felt before. Hunger can lead to failure. Eating the right balance of nutrients can ensure that hunger does not occur. When calories are reduced, every calorie counts. Foods high in dietary fat are higher in calories but not necessarily nutrition. Nevertheless, they have a place in a weight-loss plan. Eliminating them completely can lead to cravings and hunger, because they slow down the digestion of other foods. The same is true regarding eating lean protein that is lower in calories. Because protein increases satiation, a meal with protein can help you feel full and satisfied until your next meal. Plus, studies show that eating more protein while trying to reduce body fat protects against muscle loss. Another nutrient that helps with satiation is fiber. Including slightly more lean protein, fiber-rich carbohydrate sources, and a bit of healthy fat at every meal is the recipe for healthy and successful weight loss. Remember, you should not eliminate food groups. Each nutrient has a place in the meal plan and should be included. Modify; do not eliminate or restrict.

I have been analyzing diets for almost 20 years, and I can tell you it is hard enough to meet the nutrition needs of a growing adolescent athlete who does not restrict, let alone one who does. Take the paleo diet, for example. It promotes eating many healthy foods such as vegetables, lean protein, nuts, and seeds, but it restricts foods such as grains and dairy that are great sources of vitamin D, calcium, and B vitamins. Following a restrictive plan without proper knowledge of how to obtain these needed nutrients can be dangerous and result in injuries. If a diet promises quick weight loss, has a list of foods you should never eat, or sounds too good to be true, avoid it. Instead, focus on modifying your current diet and using the following strategies to reduce your overall calories.

Avoid Fried Foods

Fried foods are high in calories. Period. Replace fried chicken with grilled chicken, French fries with baked fries, and batter-dipped fish with pan-seared fish.

Choose Lean Protein

White meat (such as chicken breast) is lower in calories and fat than dark meat (chicken legs and thighs), and certain cuts of beef are leaner than others. Look for poultry that has the phrase *all white meat* and beef that is 93 percent lean or higher. Cuts of beef with the words *round* or *loin* are the lowest in fat. Remove all visible, natural fat from foods. This includes pulling the skin from raw poultry and trimming the fat from steak.

Decrease Portion Size

You can lower your energy intake by hundreds of calories per day simply by eating less of the foods you already eat. Take the amount of food that you would normally eat, but leave a quarter of it on the plate. As you begin to understand how much food is enough for you, decrease the amount of food you put on your plate. Every meal should include a healthy carbohydrate, a lean protein, and a small amount of healthy fat.

Avoid Liquid Calories

Liquids move through the stomach faster than solid foods do; therefore, they don't have the same satiety factor. Drinking calories does not satisfy hunger and generally does not provide fiber. For example, rather than orange juice, eat an orange. Avoid soda and sugar-sweetened beverages; instead, drink water or skim milk.

Recover Smart

Recovery nutrition is important for athletes, but if you are trying to lose weight, you have to make every calorie count. For example, many athletes drink chocolate milk after a workout as a recovery beverage, but if you are trying to lose weight, the chocolate syrup in the milk provides sugar without nutrients. When calories are reduced, every calorie must count. A better recovery meal would be 8 ounces (240 ml) of skim milk and a banana. This provides the same amount of carbohydrate and protein but more nutrients.

Avoid Extras

Adding toppings to foods can result in hundreds of unwanted calories. It is not necessary to completely avoid them, but be mindful. Order salad dressing on the side, top your potato with salsa instead of sour cream, and opt for cheese pizza over sausage pizza.

Replace Full Fat With Reduced Fat

I am not a fan of most fat-free products, but buying reduced-fat items can be a quick way to shave calories without eliminating the food completely. Choose skim or 1 percent over whole milk and lower-fat sour cream over full-fat sour cream, and use reduced-fat butter or margarine.

Food Rules

Eat Meals; No Grazing

I dislike the word *snack* because it conjures up visions of chips, pretzels, sweets, or a single piece of fruit. Although fruit is healthy, if you are really hungry, a single piece of fruit is not enough. Replace *snack* with *mini-meal*, and aim to eat one or two of them between regular meals. Mini-meals should contain at least two food groups and include a source of high-quality protein. Youth athletes who are reducing their calories need to make sure that the foods they eat provide good nutrition that contributes to their daily needs. They also need filling foods that will help them feel satisfied until their next meal. A few handfuls of pretzels might be enough calories, but they do not provide the protein needed to support growth or the satiety needed to prevent hunger. A better option is to reduce the number of pretzels to only one handful and pair them with half a turkey sandwich. Both are comparable in calories, but the mini-meal provides the food group combination and the protein to help with satiety. Plus, eating a mini-meal makes you feel as though you actually ate a meal and helps to prevent grazing and picking at foods in between meals.

Never Use Food as a Reward

Never, ever use food as a reward for good behavior. Healthy food nourishes the body, and including an occasional sweet treat and favorite food as part of a healthy plan teaches youngsters how to have both. Using food as a reward teaches young athletes to categorize foods as good or bad and can lead to negative feelings about food. Studies show that using tasty foods as a reward makes them more enticing to kids. Equally, making kids stay at the dinner table until they finish their vegetables makes them less interested in healthy food. Use other items as rewards for good behavior, such as books, new music downloads, or movies.

Be a Role Model

Spitting out advice is easy, but youth athletes are much more likely to do what parents and coaches do, not what they say. Nutrition is taught from an early age in the home; expecting children or teenagers to eat vegetables when parents do not is unrealistic. Parents should not tell their young

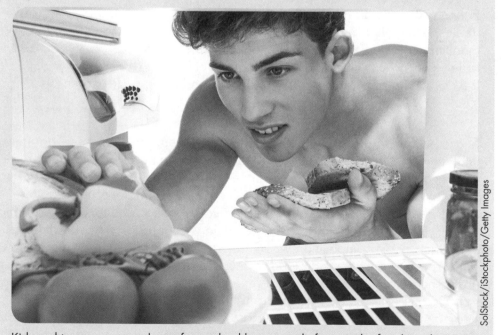

SolStock/iStockphoto/Getty Images

Kids and teenagers come home from school hungry and often eat the first thing they see that seems appealing. Parents can help young athletes eat well by making sure that the pantry and refrigerator are stocked with healthy food.

athletes how to eat right; they should show them. Coaches can do this by providing the right options for recovery or by selecting eating establishments after the game that offer healthy choices.

Make It a Family Affair

If a child needs to lose weight, it is not only the child's concern; it is the family's concern. When one child is struggling with weight, singling her out as having a problem can leave her feeling isolated and be a big blow to her self-esteem. Keep the situation positive and focus on how the family can eat better together. Family members should work together to be healthier and more physically active.

Create a Healthy Environment

You can't eat what is not in the house. If children or teenagers come home from school or sport practice hungry, they are likely to grab the first thing they see. If the cabinet is filled with chips, pretzels, and sweet treats, there is a high likelihood that is what they will choose. Telling kids not to eat those things will not work. Parents can help them be successful by getting trigger or comfort foods out of the house and filling cabinets with healthy foods and snacks that are ready to eat. This does not mean that children should be deprived of foods they like. If they really want ice cream, drive to the store and buy a small cone. Feed the craving without overindulging.

Power Down During Mealtimes

Eating right includes paying attention to what you are eating, not your electronics. Being engaged in a texting conversation or watching videos during mealtime can lead to overeating. It is hard to pay attention to hunger and satiety cues when your mind is buried in an electronic device. Power down the device, turn off the television, and focus on fueling your body properly.

Successful youth athletes are usually highly driven. That drive is what helps them excel at their sport. When they learn that building muscle or decreasing body fat could improve their performance, they might be tempted to get started right away. But changing body composition in the middle of the training or competitive season is not always ideal. As you just read, building muscle and decreasing body fat require time and attention. Encouraging youth athletes to change their body composition when they are focused on school, homework, training, and competition can lead to increased stress and result in failure. It can also negatively affect their performance. The best time to focus on changing body composition is during the transition phase of the training cycle, when the training load is lower and athletes are not focused on winning games. That does not mean that they will not benefit from learning how to eat better. Athletes should pay attention to how they fuel their bodies and understand the role nutrition plays in supporting their training and goals. Focusing on one goal at a time will ensure success.

Chapter 5

Fueling for Game Day

Chapters 2 and 3 of this book focus on the individual nutrients needed for properly fueling youth athletes. By now you should understand the role carbohydrate plays in providing energy, the need for high-quality protein for building and repairing tissues, and the important role fat plays in providing energy and satiety. You understand that what you eat every day affects how you grow, develop, feel, and perform. You are now ready to calculate your nutrition needs. But first, a quiz: Which of the following is the most important nutrition consideration for improving sport performance?

    a. What you eat the morning of an event

    b. What you eat during the event

    c. What you eat after the event

    d. What you eat every day leading up to the event

If you answered *d,* you are correct. Let's review.

What you eat every day leading up to the big day matters most because nutritional deficiencies that result in decreased performance do not happen overnight. Nor can they be corrected overnight. Take iron deficiency, for example. The fatigue that results from iron-deficiency anemia cannot be resolved by eating iron-rich foods or popping iron supplements on game day. Iron-deficiency anemia is the result of inadequate iron intake over months or years.

The same is true of macronutrients. Eating adequate protein day after day builds new muscle mass, and adequate carbohydrate intake allows you to train hard. This happens over time, not on game day. Remember, the diet that supports your training is just as important, if not more important, than what you eat the day of the event.

Keeping your body nourished and strong leading up to game day confers a competitive advantage. Now you can take it one step further. Eating for competition is all about keeping your body well fueled and well hydrated before, during, and after the event; this will give you even more of a competitive advantage. You need to start well hydrated and with glycogen-filled muscles, maintain adequate hydration throughout the activity, and then replace lost fluids and eat to start the recovery process after the event. This chapter explains how to fuel to keep your engine running at optimal capacity from the night before competition; immediately before, during, and after competition; and for days afterward. Remember, healthy hydration before, during, and after activity is the most important consideration for athletes. Combining the hydration guidelines in chapter 3 with the fueling guidelines in this chapter will result in a rock-solid sport nutrition plan.

The Evening Before Competition

Loading up on carbohydrate the evening before an athletic event is a common practice in the world of sports. Pasta parties, as they are sometimes called, start as young as sixth grade in some sports and often involve having a parent prepare a carbohydrate-rich meal for the team. One common question I get from parents is whether there is any other carbohydrate-rich meal besides pasta to feed to growing athletes. The answer is yes.

Planning a meal for the evening before a game requires first understanding the purpose of the meal. What you eat the evening before competition affects your nutritional status when you wake up the next morning. It also can affect how you feel. The goal is to go to sleep well hydrated, well fed, and satisfied but not stuffed so that you wake up feeling energized and ready to compete.

Following are a few things to consider about eating the evening before a morning competition. Table 5.1 provides the nutrient amount of a sample meal for the evening before competition.

Eat Ample Complex Carbohydrate

You won't be using the energy this meal provides until the next day, so skip the simple sugar and load up on complex carbohydrate. The aim of the meal is to fill, not overfill, muscles with glycogen. Stuffing yourself with carbohydrate can result in a stomachache and trouble sleeping, neither of which will help with sport performance. Consider the amount of carbohydrate you consume with most of your evening meals, and increase by 25 percent. It does not have to be pasta. Great alternatives are rice, quinoa, flour or corn tortillas, potatoes, sweet potatoes, pancakes, and bread.

Keep the Meal Low in Fat

Fat adds flavor, and all meals need that, but meals that are too high in fat can leave you feeling too full and can result in undereating other nutrients. You want to have plenty of room in your stomach to eat an adequate amount of carbohydrate.

Limit Fiber and Other Gas-Producing Foods

Bran cereals, beans, legumes, and cruciferous vegetables (such as broccoli, brussels sprouts, and cabbage) contribute significantly to the diet, but not at the time of competition. These foods can cause gas and temporary bloating as they work through the digestive tract—not something you want to deal with around competition.

Include Lean Protein

Although the focus is on taking in enough carbohydrate to fuel your body during competition, you still need protein and nutrients to meet your nutritional needs and to function properly. Include 3 to 4 ounces (90 to 120 g) of lean protein with the meal. Good options are lean ground beef, turkey, fish, chicken, and tofu.

Focus on Fluids

The day and evening before an event are no time to get relaxed on your fluid intake. Going to sleep well hydrated is critical to tomorrow's hydration status. Be sure to stick to your hydration schedule the day before, and go to bed well hydrated. As soon as you get up, drink water.

Avoid New Foods

Nothing that you eat around competition time should be new or experimental; that's what training is for. Stick to familiar foods that you know your body tolerates. This can be a challenge if you are traveling. You can choose plain foods at restaurants or bring your own meals. Figure 5.1 later in this chapter, the athlete's portable pantry, provides examples of foods you can take on the road.

Table 5.1 Sample Meal for the Evening Before Competition With Nutrient Amounts

	Carbohydrate (g)	Protein (g)	Fat (g)
2 whole-wheat tortillas (6 in., or 15 cm)	50	6	2
3 oz (90 g) chicken	0	20	2
1 oz (30 g) shredded cheese	0	7	9
2 tbsp (30 g) sour cream	0	0	5
1/4 sautéed pepper with onions (cooked in 1 tsp, or 5 ml, olive oil)	2	0	5
1 cup white rice, cooked	60	5	0
10 strawberries, medium	8	0	0
8 oz (240 ml) milk, skim	12	8	0
Total	132	46	23

To Carbohydrate-Load or Not to Carbohydrate-Load

Carbohydrate loading, more recently referred to as muscle glycogen supercompensation, is the practice of training muscles to store the maximal amount of glycogen in preparation for an event. In adult athletes who engage in intense, continuous endurance activity lasting longer than 90 minutes, this practice has been shown to improve performance. The practice has not been found to be beneficial in activities of shorter duration or lower intensity. There is little scientific evidence to support this practice in youth athletes. Even without the evidence, there is reason to question how beneficial it would be for this population, especially preadolescent athletes.

Young children have a limited ability to store carbohydrate and therefore may rely more on fat to fuel their activity than adults do. Although glycogen storage capacity improves as they move through adolescence, carbohydrate loading in youth athletes is not recommended. Instead, a strong emphasis should be placed on consuming at least 50 percent of daily total energy needs from carbohydrate-rich foods, because they provide energy, nutrients, and fiber. For younger athletes who participate in intensive, continuous endurance activities lasting longer than 90 minutes, refined carbohydrate products such as sport drinks, gels, and energy bars can be helpful during training and competition. Athletes should be educated on their purpose and proper use of these products.

Remember, youth athletes come in all shapes and sizes and develop at different rates. The meal eaten the evening before competition should be similar to the typical balanced meal eaten on other nights of the week, but with more of a focus on complex carbohydrate. The sample meal shown in table 5.1 can be altered to include fewer calories by decreasing the portion size of each food, but do not completely eliminate one of the foods. The same is true for athletes who require more calories. Increase the portion size of all foods, so that the balance of nutrients remains adequate and the meal supplies a variety of vitamins and minerals.

The Morning of Training or Competition

Whether the event starts at 5:00 a.m., 9:00 a.m., or 2:00 p.m., youth athletes need to eat before they compete. Eating before competing, also called competing in a fed state, has been shown to improve performance. The preworkout meal gives a competitive advantage for a variety of reasons. First, carbohydrate-rich foods and fluids help to restore liver glycogen stores after an overnight fast. This is why we stress the importance of breakfast (i.e., breaking the fast). A carbohydrate-rich meal also tops off muscle glycogen stores, prevents hunger, and provides a mental boost while entering competition.

One of the problems I see as a sport dietitian is oversimplified eating advice that assumes that all athletes have the same goals, level of training, and type and duration of activity. This is simply not true. What an athlete needs before a competition and what a fitness enthusiast needs before a 30-minute spin class differ markedly. A long-distance runner's needs before a workout are very different from a bodybuilder's needs before an on-stage competition. If you want to know which preworkout meal is best for you, base it on you. Remember that most preworkout fueling recommendations are meant to improve your performance—help you train harder, compete better, and come out a champion. If you are reading this book, I assume that you want to win. The recom-

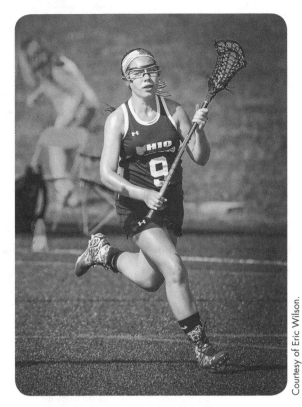

Athletes need an adequate pregame meal to keep them fueled, hydrated, and energized throughout the entire game.

Courtesy of Eric Wilson.

mendations in this chapter are for athletes in the training and competition phase of their seasons. If your goal is to change body composition, refer to chapter 4, which discusses decreasing body fat and gaining lean muscle mass.

So what does the perfect preworkout meal look like? Research on how much carbohydrate youth athletes need to eat in the hours before competition does not exist, although we can make some assumptions based on research on adults. Remember that youth athletes develop at different rates, and the amount of food they eat varies incredibly from one athlete to another. Following are some general nutrient guidelines:

- *Carbohydrate.* Focus on carbohydrate sources such as whole-grain breads, pasta, tortillas, rice, cereals, fruits, and vegetables. Eating carbohydrate-rich foods before exercise can supply energy and maximize muscle glycogen stores. The more time you have before the competition, the more complex carbohydrate you can have. The closer you are to competition, the more simple carbohydrate you should have. The timing also influences whether to choose solid fuel or liquid fuel. Athletes who find it difficult to tolerate solid foods should focus on liquid fuel. (Chapter 10 provides liquid-fuel recipes, and chapter 11 provides solid-fuel recipes.)

- *Protein.* The preevent meal should contain a small to moderate amount of protein. The closer you are to competition, the less protein you should consume.
- *Fat and fiber.* Keep the preworkout meal low in fat and fiber. Meals high in fat and fiber take longer to digest, which may cause fullness and other gastrointestinal (GI) issues such as nausea, bloating, cramping, and general discomfort.
- *Hydrating foods.* Hydrating foods are great for providing additional fluid. Fruits, vegetables, smoothies, and yogurt are good options.
- *Salty foods.* For long-duration activities, or when exercising in extreme conditions, salty foods help prevent sodium depletion. Good choices are chicken broth, pickles, olives, and pretzels.

Some of my clients have reported that they prefer to compete on an empty stomach. Here is what I say to that: If your goal is to burn calories or lose weight and athletic performance is not your concern, go for it. But if your goal is to get faster and stronger, build muscle, perform better, and win, you need preworkout fuel. However, I do not recommend competing on a full stomach. The closer you are to the competition, the less food you should consume. The more time you have before competing, the more food you can consume. Higher-intensity workouts require more time for digestion. If you know your stomach

Making Weight

Youth athletes who participate in weight-class sports often believe that they must restrict fluid and food intake to make weight. Such voluntary restriction is traditionally seen in sports such as rowing, wrestling, boxing, and mixed martial arts, but it does not stop there. Athletes who participate in any sport emphasizing thinness, leanness, and competing at the lowest weight possible should be considered at risk for unhealthy weight loss practices and understand the risks. Voluntary dehydration practices include intentionally restricting fluids; using laxatives or diuretics; spitting; and using saunas, steam rooms, or rubber suits (also called sauna suits) to increase sweat loss.

Restricting fluid and food can be harmful to the health and performance of any athlete and is not recommended. Dehydration and underfueling decrease performance; therefore, taking in the proper amounts of fluid and fuel should be a priority even in weight-class sports. Because youth athletes in these sports may be tempted to participate in unhealthy practices, they need guidance and education on healthy weight-control alternatives. They may benefit from choosing liquid fuel over solid fuel, because liquids produce a lower stool residue, thereby minimizing immediate weight gain.

can't handle solid food before a workout, opt for a smoothie or sport drink for the added carbohydrate (see chapter 10 for liquid-fuel recipes). Even within the same sport and position, athletes differ in terms of the type and amount of food they can tolerate before exercise. Practice preworkout fueling until you learn what works for you. The following are some fueling recommendations based on the amount of time before competition.

Three to Four Hours Before Training or Competition

If you have three to four hours before your competition, you have plenty of time to eat, digest, absorb, and metabolize a healthy balanced meal. Of course, you should also stay focused on your hydration schedule (refer to chapter 3 for specifics on hydrating before, during, and after activity). Moreover, you need to eat the right foods. Table 5.2 is an example of a healthy precompetition breakfast for both female and male athletes. The amount of food you eat should be based on your day-to-day meal plan (you can calculate this using the information in chapters 2 and 3). As mentioned, estimating the needs of a youth athlete based on chronological age is difficult, because developmental age is the main influencer.

Table 5.2 Nutrient Amounts of a Sample Meal Three to Four Hours Before Competition

Female adolescent athlete			
	Carbohydrate (g)	Protein (g)	Fat (g)
2 frozen waffles	27	5	6
2 tbsp (30 ml) syrup	25		
2 oz (60 g) ham steak		11	3
1/2 banana	13		
3 walnut halves, crushed			4
8 oz (240 ml) milk, skim	12	8	
Total (~525 calories)	77	24	13
Male adolescent athlete			
3 frozen waffles	39	8	9
3 tbsp (45 ml) syrup	40		
3-4 oz (90-120 g) ham steak		17	4
1 banana, medium	27		
6 walnut halves, crushed	1	1	8
8 oz (240 ml) milk, skim	12	8	
Total (~800 calories)	119	34	21

Because this meal is consumed three to four hours before competition, it may be necessary to top off muscle glycogen stores immediately before activity. The additional fuel and fluids needed to support your body in competition are provided in the section on what to eat immediately before competition.

One and a Half to Two and a Half Hours Before Training or Competition

As you get closer to the time of competition, the amount of food you eat should decrease, but the balance and composition of the meals should be similar. You still need to nourish your body and provide fuel for your working muscles, but you do not want to eat so much that you have undigested food in your stomach when the competition starts. The main focus of this preworkout mini-meal is carbohydrate, the fuel your muscles will use during activity. As mentioned earlier, some athletes prefer liquid nutrition over solids precompetition, especially as nerves and anxiety begin to take over.

Don't panic if your preworkout meal is not as balanced as recommended here. If you find it difficult to eat anything solid, or find certain foods problematic, avoid them. A simple sport drink or other liquid nutrition source can provide some carbohydrate for your working muscles to use during competition. If eating solids before activity is not a problem for you, aim for about 250 calories and 40 to 60 grams of easily digested carbohydrate as well as a little fat and protein to prevent you from getting hungry during competition. Table 5.3 lists the nutrient amounts of a few common balanced mini-meals that you can experiment with before your training. Remember that we all need differ-

Table 5.3 Mini-Meals for One and a Half to Two and a Half Hours Before Competition With Nutrient Amounts

	Calories	Carbohydrate (g)	Protein (g)	Fat (g)
1/2 turkey sandwich; 1 orange	200	33	14	2
Fruit yogurt; 1 tsp (5 g) nuts, crushed; 2 tsp (10 g) fruit, dried	207	38	5	3
3/4 cup cereal; 6 oz (180 ml) milk, skim	200	40	9	1
granola bar, crunchy; banana	225	40	4	5
Nut butter and jelly sandwich (1 tbsp, or 15 g, peanut butter; 1 tsp, or 5 g, jelly); 1/4 cup grapes	280	40	11	10
4 fig bars	220	44	2	5

Table 5.4 Carbohydrate Food Suggestions for Immediately Before Competition

	Calories	Carbohydrate (g)
1 banana, medium	105	27
4 apricots, dried	80	20
20 oz (600 ml) sport drink	158	40
1 orange, medium	80	19
2 rice cakes	120	24
1 oz (30 g) pretzels, salted	101	23

ent amounts of food, so adjust your portions based on your total daily needs. See chapter 8 to learn how to create a personal meal skeleton based on your personal goals and training.

Immediately Before Training or Competition

How close to my competition can I eat or drink? I get asked this question often, and my answer is always the same: It depends.

Although having a healthy, balanced meal three to four hours before training or competition is ideal, it is not always possible. High school swimmers, for example, often have to be at the pool by 5:30 a.m. for practice. When training or a competition is early in the morning, the meal eaten the night before is critical, and eating something before activity is necessary, too. There are no concrete guidelines for what to eat immediately before activity. Some youth athletes tolerate solid food quite well right before activity; others do not. Consuming easily digested, simple carbohydrate will likely be better tolerated than complex carbohydrate. Liquid fuel may be easier to tolerate than solid fuel. Training or competing at a high intensity with food in your stomach puts you at high risk for nausea. Therefore, the greater the intensity of your training or sport, the more time you need between eating and activity.

Some athletes have increased anxiety immediately before competition and simply cannot eat. The last thing you want to do is eat or drink something if you are filled with stress and anxiety. If you know this about yourself, focus on eating a balanced meal three to four hours before your competition; then sip a sport drink in the hour before activity. Table 5.4 lists some sources of simple carbohydrate to top off glycogen stores immediately before activity.

During Training or Competition

A study published in the *International Journal of Sport Nutrition and Exercise Metabolism* (Baker et al., 2014) showed that carbohydrate fueling during activity was the most common shortfall in 29 athletes ages 14 to 19. As a sport dietitian, that doesn't surprise me. When I interview youth athletes on what they eat and drink during activity, the most common response is water. Although sport drinks are sometimes reported, athletes are rarely able to report exactly how much sport drink they consume. Longer-distance endurance athletes seem to be the most tuned in to how much they consume. Whatever the activity, if it lasts longer than one hour, water is most likely not enough. So what is enough? Giving specific recommendations is tricky, especially for youth athletes. Studies on how much fluid and carbohydrate adults should consume during activity are widely available, but that is not the case for adolescents. The guidance and recommendations given here are based on adult studies combined with my experience working with youth athletes.

Research on adults reveals that consuming carbohydrate during activity that lasts longer than one hour can delay the onset of fatigue, help maintain blood glucose levels, and ultimately benefit performance. Although much of the focus in this area has been on endurance activity, more recent research has shown benefits in stop-and-go sports such as tennis, basketball, and football. Given that adolescents have higher nutritional needs than adults and are at greater risk for dehydration, fluid and carbohydrate intake during activity is recommended.

Consuming carbohydrate during activity has some benefit, but the body is limited in how much it can handle during exercise. Knowing this has allowed sport scientists to make fueling recommendations for adult athletes in grams of carbohydrate rather than by body weight. The recommendation is to consume 30 to 60 grams of carbohydrate per hour during endurance and intermittent, high-intensity exercise lasting from 60 to 90 minutes. Although this recommendation is for adult athletes, it can be used as a guide for younger athletes.

Easy-to-digest carbohydrate sources such as energy bars, fruit, and sport drinks are good foods for long-duration activity (remember, no more than 60 grams per hour). Table 5.5 lists fluids and foods that meet these guidelines. Remember not to try a new food or fluid on the day of a competition. Practice, practice, practice.

It is worth mentioning that some products specifically formulated for consumption during activity (e.g., gels, beans, chews), although providing carbohydrate and electrolytes, do not contain fluid. If these products are your fuel of choice, you will need to drink enough water to maintain a healthy fluid status.

Table 5.5   Carbohydrate Food and Fluid Suggestions During Competition

	Carbohydrate (g)
20 oz (600 ml) sport drink (no more than 8 oz, or 240 ml, every 15 min)	40
3 rice cakes (3)	36
1 banana, medium	27
Sport nutrition energy bar (varies by brand and size)	47
2 gel packs	50
28 sport beans	50

Consuming these products without sufficient water can lead to dehydration, GI distress, and other potentially dangerous health consequences. Sport drinks, on the other hand, are more diluted and have the electrolytes, carbohydrate, and fluid all in one product. If you drink sport drinks in addition to using gels, beans, or chew, you risk consuming too much carbohydrate. The result is GI distress, including nausea, stomach cramping, and diarrhea that you won't soon forget. Make sure to calculate your carbohydrate intake per hour.

GI distress can occur for several reasons, not all of which are related to nutrition. However, if it is a nutrition issue, a few simple tweaks in the meal plan can result in big improvements. Studies have shown that exercise performance is improved with feedings of glucose and fructose during activity. However, fructose used alone was associated with complaints of GI distress. Fructose, the natural sugar found in foods such as fruit and honey, is absorbed more slowly than glucose and requires an extra step before muscles can use it. Certain fruits are rich in concentrated fructose and, when consumed alone in high amounts, can be problematic. In most cases, it is not the fruit that causes GI distress; it is the amount of fructose consumed within a certain time frame. Using a combination of carbohydrate sources during activity (glucose with fructose, or glucose with fructose and sucrose) can decrease the risk of GI distress. Studies in adult athletes also show that using multiple transportable carbohydrate, compared with a single carbohydrate, may reduce fatigue and improved performance. The same may be true for youth athletes.

An additional concern for youth athletes who choose prepared sport nutrition products is added ingredients. Some products contain caffeine or other herbal ingredients that can pose health risks, especially when exercising in the heat or other extreme conditions. The safest and smartest foods and fluids to consume during activity are those that are tried and true, that your body is familiar with, and that you know work well.

After Training or Competition

The food consumed immediately after training or competition is referred to as the recovery meal. All youth athletes who participate in exhaustive activity should begin the refueling process within 30 minutes after activity. This meal is even more important for those who are preparing for another competition the same day or the next day.

Although *recovery nutrition* is a popular term, there is a lot of confusion about which foods should be eaten right after activity. It is well accepted that carbohydrate is the most critical component of the recovery meal; however, many athletes are convinced that protein is more important. To understand what makes an ideal recovery snack, you have to understand what is happening to the body after exercise and how what you eat affects how you recover. After a hard training session or competition, your muscles are depleted of glycogen. The purpose of the recovery meal is to replenish your glycogen stores so that your muscles are ready to go for your next exercise session. Properly

Michelle

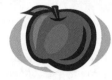

Michelle, a 16-year-old distance runner, was referred to me by her high school track coach, who had heard me speak at a local seminar about GI distress in runners. Michelle's chief complaint was that she got diarrhea whenever she ran more than 8 miles (13 km). She was worried about her long-distance running career because her symptoms got worse as she increased her daily mileage. She started to wonder whether she should stick to shorter distances, as she had in previous years. Before our appointment, I had her keep a seven-day food journal as well as track her exercise and symptoms.

Michelle was at an appropriate weight for her sport, and, according to her food journal, her total nutrition intake appeared adequate. Like most long-distance runners, she consumed a large percentage of her calories from carbohydrate sources, including lots of fruits, vegetables, and whole grains, and she appeared to eat sufficient protein and fat. We discussed how her nutrition differed on her off days, short-run days, and long-run days. Michelle understood the importance of fueling before, during, and after her training, but admitted that she included food and fluid only during long runs. She denied the use of any commercially prepared sport products, such as gels, beans, and chomps, because she found them too sweet. She preferred water over sport drink to meet her hydration needs. During her run she would consume raisins because she liked them, they were easy to carry, and they seemed to agree with her system.

After reviewing her journal, symptoms, and activity, I concluded that her day-to-day nutrition was adequate and included a wonderful variety of healthy foods. Michelle loved fruits and vegetables and fueled her longer runs with raisins rather than any engineered foods. She was unsure of how much carbohydrate she was consuming from the fruit and admitted that she didn't worry about it because it was a whole food. Raisins are a high-fructose fruit, and I suspected that Michelle was simply eating too much for her intestinal tract to handle during her run. She agreed to try a different fuel source during her long-distance running—a combination of raisins and liquid fuel. Because traditional sport drinks were too sweet for her, she made her own drink using one of the homemade recipes from chapter 10. Reducing the amount of raisins helped, and Michelle's GI symptoms resolved. She was back to running longer distances without having diarrhea. She also reported an improvement in her performance. Maybe it was because she was feeling better, or maybe it was because she was using a variety of carbohydrate sources on her long runs.

Table 5.6 Recovery Snack Suggestions for Immediately After Training or Competition

	Calories	Carbohydrate (g)	Protein (g)
12 oz (360 ml) chocolate milk	200	40	11
Chocolate peanut butter protein smoothie (see recipe in chapter 10); 1/2 cup applesauce	290	41	18
3/4 cup cereal with 8 oz (240 ml) skim milk, 1 tbsp (15 g) raisins	220	43	11
6 oz flavored Greek yogurt with 1 tbsp (15 g) honey, 1/4 cup blueberries, 12 oz (360 ml) sport drink	290	58	17
Nut butter and jelly sandwich (1 tbsp, or 15 g, peanut butter, 1 tsp, or 5 g, jelly); 1 kiwi	290	42	12
1/2 turkey sandwich; 1 banana	230	43	14

refueling after daily training sessions leads to good recovery, leaving you feeling well and prepared for your next exercise session.

For youth athletes who have multiple trainings or competitions in the same day, carbohydrate consumption should begin immediately after activity. Glycogen repletion occurs faster within the 30 minutes or so after exercise. Refueling during this small window begins the recovery process and gives athletes the best chance at beginning the next session with glycogen-filled muscles. The next section on fueling between competitions has more information.

In addition to carbohydrate, a small amount of protein in recovery snacks and meals may promote muscle tissue repair and protein balance. The recommendations for recovery nutrition should be based on the athlete's developmental age and the type and intensity of training. Youth athletes should aim to consume a minimum of 40 grams of carbohydrate and a minimum of 10 grams of protein in the recovery meal. Remember, carbohydrate is the most important nutrient to consume. A full meal should be consumed within two hours of the recovery snack. Table 5.6 shows examples of balanced recovery snacks and their nutrient contents.

Between Two Competitions

When my son was a competitive swimmer, I volunteered to work the concession stand. I was in disbelief at the choices. The menu consisted of doughnuts, candy, toaster pastries, walking tacos, macaroni and cheese, and soft pretzels. Swim meets last for hours, and many athletes rely on the foods sold at

Eating On the Go

Traveling with or without a team is part of the fun, but it can also add challenges in terms of sticking to a healthy meal plan. As a youth athlete, you do not always have control over where the bus stops after a game or what foods and fluids will be available. Today, most restaurants (even fast-food establishments) offer something that fits within the guidelines for before- and after-competition meals. Here are a few examples of meals to order in a restaurant:

- Grilled chicken breast with baked potato, vegetable, and dinner roll
- Chicken or fish fajitas with rice and vegetables
- Pasta and chicken in a plain tomato or marinara sauce
- Grilled chicken sandwich with a side salad and applesauce
- Turkey club, baked potato, and fruit cup

Situations can arise that present challenges for finding the right fuel, such as traveling to other states, especially those with different food cultures. Some teams have parents cook before a competition, and some parent may cook things you do not like. Your best defense is to pack a portable pantry, a gym bag or cooler filled with easy, convenient, often shelf-stable foods that you can take with you as a last resort. Remember that you are responsible for your own sport nutrition plan. If you want to eat right, you need to be prepared. The sidebar Athlete's Portable Pantry shows foods you can use to build your own portable pantry.

concession stands for their fuel. Many high school or youth athletic clubs use the money made at the concessions to support the club. Like it or not, doughnuts make the club more money than fresh fruit, and they are likely here to stay. My point is that relying on the food available at sporting events is not a good idea. If you want to be sure you have the right food, pack your own foods and fluids for competition day.

Fueling for back-to-back competitions can look like one of the following:

- Eating and drinking between two or three events at the same competition
- Fueling for a morning game and an evening game in the same day
- Eating and drinking to fuel for a tournament, such as a Friday evening game, a Saturday morning game, and then a Sunday morning game

Each of the preceding scenarios requires additional nutrition attention, but the principles already discussed apply as well. When determining the best thing to eat between two competitions or events, the most important consideration is how much time you have. Consider Luke, who has a Saturday morning swim meet and is to report on deck at 7:30 a.m. He will be competing in three events: the 200-meter freestyle, 100-meter butterfly, and 400-meter medley relay. His first event is expected to be at 9:30 a.m., the second around 10:30 a.m., and the last not until about 12:30 p.m. What should Luke eat to fuel his swimming?

Because his first event is not until 9:30, Luke has plenty of time to eat a healthy, balanced meal before leaving home, but he will need to pack fuel to keep his glycogen stores topped off between his events. Because he has only one hour between his first two events, he should focus on quick-digesting carbohydrates that will be out of his stomach before his next event. Following are a few examples of quick-digesting carbohydrate sources when there is less than an hour between events:

- Sport drink
- Low-fat, low-fiber energy bar
- Banana
- Graham crackers
- Gel, chews, or sport beans
- Fig bars

Table 5.7 gives an overview of eating for back-to-back bouts of exercise.

Table 5.7 Fuel Timing for Back-to-Back Exercise Bouts

Timing	Table reference
Evening before competition	Table 5.1. Extra focus on carbohydrate.
Three to four hours before competition	Table 5.2. Consume low-fat and low-fiber foods; focus on carbohydrate and fluids.
One and a half to two and a half hours before competition	Table 5.3
Immediately before competition	Table 5.4. Top off glycogen stores with easily digested carbohydrate sources.
During competition	Table 5.5
Immediately after competition	Table 5.6. Consume a recovery snack within 30 minutes of activity.
Three to four hours before the next competition	Table 5.1. Consume this meal as close to the end of the last competition as possible.
One and a half to two and a half hours before the next competition	Table 5.2. May need to include additional fluids to start as well hydrated as possible.
Multiple events within the same competition	Table 5.3. Consume simple, easily digested carbohydrate sources; portions will vary.

Athlete's Portable Pantry

Carbohydrate
- Microwavable rice pouch
- Dried fruits
- Raw fruits
- Apple sauce cups
- Bread, bagels, rice cakes, crackers
- Oatmeal

Protein
- String cheese
- Tuna pouches
- Beef jerky
- Canned chicken
- Greek yogurt

Fats
- Nuts
- Nut butter
- Seeds

These can be used to make trail mix

Fluids
- Bottled water
- Bottled sports drink
- Shelf-stable white or chocolate milk

Game day is not the time to experiment with new foods or fluids. What you eat before, during, and after competition should be calculated and practiced. It is not the time to eat more or try less to see what happens. The most prepared athletes have practiced their food and fluid regimens many times during training.

Chapter 6

Understanding Supplements

In 1997, I was the nutritionist at Gold's Gym in Flemington, New Jersey. I ran a 12-week nutrition program helping athletes and active people change their body composition. As a young nutritionist right out of college, I was eager to share my nutrition knowledge and teach my clients the influence food choices have on how they feel, look, and perform. I couldn't wait to answer questions on what foods to eat. Instead, I got a lot of questions about what supplements to take.

Fast-forward to today. In all aspects of my work (counseling, speaking, writing, and media consulting), the most common sport nutrition–related questions I get are about dietary supplements and protein. Heavy marketing of these products makes them popular, but that does not mean that they are right for youth athletes. Recommending dietary supplements for youth athletes without any evidence of safety or efficacy, or proper dosing guidelines, is potentially dangerous and irresponsible, but that won't stop teenagers from being tempted. The emphasis on muscularity in the adolescent population is greater than ever. Teens are not necessarily interested in what the science shows, nor do they care about how supplements could negatively affect their health. That's why parents, coaches, and trainers must be knowledgeable about the safety, efficacy, and reality of the industry. The potential lure of supplement abuse is real and, quite frankly, scary.

This chapter offers a glimpse into the latest research on a variety of popular ergogenic aids, including dietary supplements and other performance-enhancing products. But this list is far from all inclusive. In addition to what the limited studies and nationwide surveys show as the popular dietary supplements among teenagers and youth athletes, I include the supplements that I see and hear youth athletes discussing. I also called on some of my colleagues (sport dietitians, athletic trainers, and coaches) to share the dietary supplements they see being used or discussed. This information will prepare you to talk about a variety of dietary supplements, from beneficial products such as protein powders, sport drinks, and multivitamins to products with hidden and well-documented dangers, such as human growth hormone (HGH) and anabolic steroids. The information in this chapter gets a bit technical. Stay with me as I try to help you understand the research and rationale for and reality of what's happening in the world of dietary supplements.

What Are Supplements?

The legal definition of *dietary supplement,* according to the U.S. Food and Drug Administration (FDA), is an ingredient intended to add nutritional value to the diet. The ingredient may be a vitamin, mineral, herb, botanical, amino acid, metabolite, constituent, concentrate, extract, or a combination of any of these (National Institutes of Health, Office of Dietary Supplements 1994). Dietary supplements come in a variety of forms, including pills, chews, liquids, and tablets. Some, such as multivitamins, are commonly recommended to help ensure that daily nutrition needs are met. In the case of known nutrient deficiencies, individual vitamins and minerals (such as iron and vitamin D) can be prescribed to restore levels back to normal. Weight-loss products, diet pills, and stimulants also fall under the umbrella of dietary supplements, in addition to some products marketed directly to athletes to improve athletic performance or build muscle in the hope of being bigger, stronger, and more energized. These nutritional supplements targeted directly to athletes are often referred to as ergogenic aids.

An ergogenic aid, in the context of sport, is any technique or substance used for the purpose of enhancing performance. Using that definition, the technique of carbohydrate loading and products such as protein powders, muscle builders, preworkout shakes, energy bars, and sport drinks are considered ergogenic aids. Also included are illegal and unsafe products such as HGH and anabolic steroids, which can cause serious, irreversible health consequences and even death.

Understanding the Supplement Industry

The supplement industry is booming. Americans spent $32.5 billion on dietary supplements in 2012, which was a 7.5 percent increase over their purchases in 2011. According to a survey conducted by the Council for Responsible Nutrition (CRN) in 2014, approximately 68 percent of American adults used dietary supplements; approximately 50 percent reported regular use.

One reason for the growth in supplement use is a shift in the demographics of users of these products. Those looking to lose weight and build muscle are not the only ones seeking dietary supplements; these products are growing in popularity among the general public. Today, it seems there is a pill, potion, or powder that can solve any problem. Or at least that is what the industry wants you to believe. Supplement companies want to sell their products, and doing so means finding a way to get your attention. In the world of sport supplements, attention-getting messages often come in the form of tempting testimonials and irresistible claims often by professional athletes whom teenagers admire.

Dietary supplements are marketed as an easy way to enhance athletic performance, lose weight, build muscle, increase metabolism, and feel energized. This seemingly quick fix is surely attractive to youth athletes who want to succeed, especially in today's sport culture. Teenage athletes report increased pressure to win not only from coaches but also from parents. Peer pressure from teammates also contributes to the risk of supplement abuse.

The industry itself still poses risks. Most of my clients are shocked when I explain that nutritional supplements are not regulated by the FDA in the same way that drugs are. They fall under the Dietary Supplement Health and Education Act of 1994 (DSHEA), which states that the FDA is responsible for taking action against adulterated misbranded products only after they reach the market and a complaint is filed. No evidence of efficacy or safety is required before a product hits the shelf. Manufacturers are responsible for evaluating the safety and labeling of their own products before marketing them to ensure that they meet all of the standards. The problem? Not all manufacturers are testing their raw ingredients for purity the way you might expect them to, and the companies that do are often shocked by what they find.

A survey was conducted in 2007 by Informed-Choice, which describes itself as "a quality assurance program for sports nutrition, suppliers to the sports nutrition industry, and supplement manufacturing facilities." The survey of 58 supplement samples from various retail outlets reported that 11 percent contained stimulants not listed on the label. Some of the products contained steroids. Even companies that voluntarily chose to have their products tested have been surprised to find banned substances identified. Products that are manufactured in the United States may use raw ingredients from China, and cross-contamination, even when not intentional, is a reality. Botanical, or plant-based, supplements are especially risky because they may contain low levels of a banned substance naturally. Unfortunately, this can damage a sport career.

In 2013, the FDA reported that an outbreak of hepatitis that had struck at least 72 people in 16 states was traced to a tainted supplement. In 2014, researchers investigated 14 dietary supplements and identified in some of them a synthetic stimulant never tested in humans (1,3-dimethylbutylamine, or DMBA). DMBA is similar to the pharmaceutical stimulant 1,3 dimethylamylamine (DMAA), which was recently banned by the FDA (Pieter et al., 2015). The products found to contain DMBA were marketed to improve athletic performance, increase weight loss, and enhance brain function. The products were sold at popular vitamin stores, ones I can almost guarantee you have heard of.

In 2015, the New York attorney general accused four major retailers of selling fraudulent and potentially dangerous herbal supplements after authorities found that four of five products did not contain any of the herbs listed on the label. Instead, the pills contained cheap fillers such as powdered rice, houseplants, and in some cases products that could be dangerous to those with allergies.

Fuel Focus

Jake

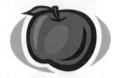

Jake, a 16-year-old hockey player, came to see me complaining of fatigue. "I just can't make it through my games without feeling tired," he said. He was interested in learning what he could take to give him more energy. He had read that vitamin B_{12} had something to do with energy production, and he thought he might need a supplement.

After reviewing his food journal, I wasn't so convinced. Jake was a growing, active athlete, and he ate lots of food. What was missing was fluid. As we started talking, Jake admitted that he probably didn't drink enough, but he didn't think that was the problem. In fact, he explained, "I usually don't get thirsty until the third period."

I suspected that dehydration was causing Jake's fatigue. I assessed his hydration status by having him keep a fluid journal for a few days. He calculated his changes in body weight, evaluated his urine color, rated his thirst, and tracked his overall feelings of fatigue. In the meantime, I assessed his basic fluid needs (using the dietary reference intakes, or DRIs), and we determined his sweat rate.

We concluded that Jake was getting dehydrated. He needed to learn the importance of hydration and the warning signs and symptoms of dehydration. He also needed a hydration plan. Once he understood the importance of hydration and started to practice his plan, his energy levels improved and he saw immediate performance benefits.

My point is that the quality and purity of many dietary supplements on the market are questionable. What you read on the bottle is not always what you get. Read labels, but be skeptical. If you do make the choice to use a supplement, look for products that are third-party certified or verified. Certification from an independent, accredited third party helps confirm that products contain only the ingredients and quantities shown on the label without potentially harmful levels of impurities. NSF Certified for Sport, for example, screens for more than 200 banned or prohibited substances such as hormones, stimulants, steroids, and narcotics as well as diuretics and masking agents. Informed-Choice (www.informed-choice.org) is another organization that tests the dietary supplements and ingredients of manufacturers that participate in their program.

Another resource is ConsumerLab.com, a privately held company that purchases supplements on the open market. Its research group analyzes the quantity, identity, and purity of key ingredients and evaluates other issues of product quality. They publish reports on nearly every popular supplement and name-brand product on their website. You can subscribe to their service to receive information on a variety of products, including multivitamins, protein powders, popular energy bars. The yearly subscription does have a small fee, but it may be worth it to gather the latest information on the safety, purity, and quality of products you may be considering.

Common Supplements Used by High School Athletes

I know what I see, but I also interviewed a few of my colleagues who are experts in the field to compare our experiences. As it turns out, we are all on the same page in terms of what's popular. Among high school athletes, the most popular supplements seem to be protein powder, preworkout products, creatine products, and energy drinks. Youth athletes openly admit to using these products and see nothing wrong with doing so. Let's review what the research shows.

Studies looking at usage are limited, and the little data we have vary. For one, the criteria for what is considered a dietary supplement vary from survey to survey. What one study considers an ergogenic aid, another study does not include. A 2006 article published in the journal *Pediatrics* (Calfee and Fasdale, 2006) summarized the literature on popular ergogenic drugs and supplements used by youth athletes. Because the researchers looked only at illicit substances or compounds marketed as dietary supplements, they did not study protein powders or individual vitamin and mineral supplements, which are popular with youth athletes. Their report showed that youth athletes used anabolic-androgenic steroids, steroid precursors, growth hormone, creatine, and ephedra alkaloids.

In 2007, a survey review revealed very different results: Whereas one study reported creatine and caffeine as top supplements used by adolescents, other studies reported protein powders, energy drinks, and sport drink at the top of the list (McDowell, 2007). The most popular supplements reported were likely so different because they included vitamins, minerals, and herbal products as well as what many consider sport supplements in the investigator's reports. More recently, a group of researchers set out to determine the dietary supplements American children and adolescents use specifically to enhance sport performance. Most of the participants who reported using supplements used multivitamins or mineral combinations followed by fish oil and omega-3 supplements, creatine, and fiber (Evans Jr. et al., 2012).

My point? Determining the most common ergogenic aids used by youth athletes is difficult not only because of the mixed research but also because when teenagers are aware of the potential dangers of a product, they are less likely to admit to taking it. And the products that youth athletes hide are often the ones that pose the biggest risks.

Survey data from 2,793 diverse adolescents (mean age of 14.4) showed that muscle-enhancing behaviors were common among both boys and girls (Eisenburg et al., 2012). Protein supplements or shakes were used by 35 percent of the teenagers in the study. More alarming is the fact that anabolic steroid use was reported in 5.9 percent of boys and 4.6 percent of girls. This use of muscle-enhancing supplements is much higher than what was reported in previous years.

The 2013 Partnership Attitude Tracking Study supports the upward trend of steroid use in teens; it reported an increase from 5 percent in 2009 to 7 percent in 2013. And steroids are not the only performance-enhancing drugs reported by teenagers; equally alarming was that both boys and girls reported using HGH without a prescription. The results showed a significant increase—a doubling—in the use of HGH among teens. According to the survey, 11 percent of teens in grades 9 through 12 reported having used synthetic growth hormone at some point without a prescription. That is up from just 5 percent in the 2012 study. The 2013 study showed a strong correlation between the use of synthetic HGH and the use of steroids. Currently, one in five teens (21 percent) believes it is easy to obtain steroids.

Let's dig a little deeper into performance-enhancing drugs as well as others that youth athletes may show interest in. Some of this information can get technical. My goal is not to confuse you with scientific terms but instead to educate you. Understanding how supplements work and the rationale behind them will empower you to have conversations about them with youth athletes.

Steroids

Anabolic steroids are artificially produced hormones that mimic the work of androgens, the male sex hormones in the body. Although there are a few appropriate medical uses for them, they are illegal without a prescription and banned for use in sports. Some young athletes may be tempted to take steroids illegally because of their testosterone effects, such as increasing muscle mass and strength. The long list of serious side effects reveals their danger.

Anabolic steroids are usually taken orally or injected into the muscles, although some can be applied to the skin as a cream, gel, or patch. The dangers of steroid use range from less medically serious effects such as acne, oily skin, and excess hair growth to very serious effects such as liver damage, fluid retention, heart disease, and stroke (or worse). In adolescent athletes, the use of steroids can disrupt normal growth and development, causing stunted growth, accelerated puberty changes, and abnormal sexual development.

If you think the use of steroids in youth athletes is not a concern, think again. According to research from the Taylor Hooton Foundation, over 1.5 million teens have admitted to using steroids, and the median age for first-time use is 15. And it's not just boys; teen girls are the fastest-growing group of new users. Forty percent of high school seniors say steroids are easy to obtain. And, as if steroid use is not dangerous enough, research suggests that adolescents who abuse steroids are more likely to participate in other risky behaviors. If youth athletes are tempted to try or use steroids, they are likely doing so in private. Parents, coaches, and other influential adults should be aware of the signs and symptoms of steroid abuse in teens and have a plan in place if they suspect abuse.

Human Growth Hormone

Human growth hormone (HGH) is a naturally occurring hormone that plays an important role in the growth and development of adolescents, including the growth of muscles and bones. In the late 1980s, synthetic growth hormone was developed and later approved by the FDA. HGH injections are approved, with a prescription, for treating short stature or slow growth resulting from a medical condition. Athletes may be tempted to use HGH to build muscle or improve athletic performance, although there is no evidence that it actually does so. It is often used in combination with steroids.

HGH has now become easily obtainable, illegally, over the Internet. Survey results show that experimentation with HGH by teenagers has more than doubled in the past two years (2013 Partnership Attitude Tracking Study). This finding is concerning for a number of reasons. For one, it is a health issue. HGH may interfere with the normal growth and development of an adolescent's body. Serious side effects can occur in children with normal growth who do not need growth hormone (e.g., diabetes, abnormal growth of bones and internal organs, hardening of the arteries, high blood pressure). Other side effects are blurred vision, dizziness, tingling feelings, headaches, nervousness, slow or fast heartbeat, and ear infections.

Considering that HGH is very expensive, some experts question whether the HGH supplements sold illegally actually contain synthetic HGH. Even though teens believe they are taking HGH, what they purchase may actually contain something else, perhaps something more harmful or not yet studied. Ordering performance-enhancing drugs illegally on the Internet is risky business. HGH is illegal without a prescription, banned for use in sports, and dangerous.

Prohormones

Prohormones—namely, androstenedione (andro), androstenediol, and dehydroepiandrosterone (DHEA)—are heavily marketed as testosterone-boosting supplements that are allegedly safer than anabolic steroids. Don't believe it. There is no solid evidence to support the claims that andro boosts muscle growth or improves strength. Moreover, concerns about the safety of prohormone supplements were so serious that the FDA called for a ban on all androstenedione sales. These substances are controlled and banned and can no longer be bought without a prescription.

Dietary Nitrate (Beetroot Juice)

Dietary nitrate is growing in popularity as a sport nutrition supplement. Nitrate has been encouraged for adults with cardiovascular problems because of its role in vasodilation (widening the arteries so that blood flows more easily) and other physiological effects. More recently, its potential in sport and exercise has been a hot topic. Nitric oxide, often referred to by athletes as NO, is a signaling molecule that has numerous functions in the body. The body can convert dietary nitrates (the nitrates in food) to nitrate and nitric oxide, especially during times of reduced oxygen availability, such as during higher-intensity activity. Nitrate supplementation, often in the form of beetroot juice, has been shown to assist in oxygen delivery to working muscles. More oxygen to working muscles may result in an increased ability for high-intensity exercise. Understandably, that effect is interesting to athletes who want to improve their performance.

In adult athletes, dosing protocols have been developed for use before exercise. More recently, studies are investigating how chronic dietary nitrate supplementation may support dynamic exercise. Although much more research is needed to be clear on the benefits of this approach, the research in adults looks promising. However, there is no published research on the use of beetroot juice in youth athletes and, therefore, no safety, efficacy, or dosing protocols in place.

Youth athletes should steer clear of NO supplements and instead focus on increasing their intake of dietary nitrates naturally. Vegetables such as spinach, arugula, beetroot, and celery have high concentrations of nitrate. Carrots and other root vegetables are sources, too. Because the concentration of nitrates in soil varies, it is hard to determine an exact amount for any vegetable. Organic beetroot crystals, although very expensive, are available for purchase and can be used to make smoothies or mix into other foods.

Because studies of the long-term risks associated with higher levels of nitrate are limited, caution should be taken when considering supplementation above what would be consumed through a regular balanced diet. One side effect to watch out for is beeturia, the passing of pink or red urine after consuming beetroots or foods colored with beetroot extract or pigments. This does not happen with everyone, but it can be quite alarming when not expected.

There is no evidence that increasing nitrates in the diet of youth athletes will result in improved athletic performance, but encouraging youth athletes to eat more nitrate-rich vegetables is sound advice. Beetroot juice can be made at home with a juicer, or powder or crystal forms can be purchased at health food stores. Have youth athletes try a beetroot smoothie (see chapter 11 for the recipe) before heavy training, and see if they notice a difference in their performance.

Beta-Alanine and Carnosine

When I surveyed other sport dietitians who work with youth athletes about the three most common supplements they see used in practice, preworkout supplements consistently made the list. Most youth athletes who take a preworkout supplement use beta-alanine.

Beta-alanine, both alone and combined with other supplements in a preworkout blend, has become a common dietary supplement among athletes.

It is a nonessential amino acid found naturally in the body. We can also get beta-alanine by eating foods such as chicken, beef, and pork. In the muscle, beta-alanine can be used to make carnosine. To understand the proposed rationale of taking beta- alanine, you first need to understand the role of carnosine.

During exercise, the body uses oxygen to break down glucose for energy. During high-intensity exercise, when there is not enough oxygen available, the body produces lactate. The body can convert some of that lactate to energy without using oxygen. But over time, if you maintain a high intensity of exercise, that lactate, or lactic acid, will build up faster than the body can use it. The result is a burning feeling in the muscles as well as the possibility of cramping, nausea, and weakness. At that point, exercise intensity begins to lessen.

Carnosine is a substance found naturally in the body. It appears to work as a buffering agent to control the natural rise of lactic acid in the blood. The idea is that preventing the buildup of lactic acid allows people to exercise harder and longer. Carnosine levels vary from person to person. In theory, a supplement that produces a higher concentration of muscle carnosine would benefit an athlete who produces less naturally.

So if the goal of the beta-alanine supplement is simply to increase muscle carnosine, why wouldn't an athlete just take a carnosine supplement? It is because supplementing with carnosine does not increase muscle carnosine levels. Carnosine is metabolized during digestion and never makes it to the muscle. (I know I'm getting technical, but stay with me.) This is where beta-alanine comes in. Once consumed, beta-alanine can be taken up by the muscle, where it is used to make carnosine. There is good evidence to support this. Research on adult athletes shows that supplementation with beta-alanine appears safe and does increase muscle carnosine levels.

But does that lead to improved athletic performance? And what does the science show in youth athletes?

Research in adult athletes is mixed on whether beta-alanine supplementation does anything for athletic performance. This may be because some athletes already have a high level of carnosine in their muscles and do not need further supplementation. It may also mean that it just doesn't work. There is absolutely no evidence to support its use in youth athletes. Although beta-alanine supplementation appears safe at levels investigated in the adult population, we are unsure of long-term consequences. Many of the preworkout supplements on the market are laced with other ingredients. Read labels carefully. More research is needed in order to determine whether there is any benefit to athletic performance.

Branched-Chain Amino Acids (BCAAs)

The branched-chain amino acids (BCAAs) are leucine, isoleucine, and valine. All amino acids are important for building protein, but the BCAAs are different. For one, they are burned for energy during activity, making them a potential fuel source. Other potential benefits of BCAAs are that they reduce exercise-

Table 6.1   BCAA and Leucine Contents of Popular Foods

Food	Serving	Protein (g)	BCAAs (g)	Leucine (g)
Chicken breast, cooked	4 oz (120 g)	34	6.4	2.9
Turkey breast, cooked	4 oz (120 g)	33	5.3	2.8
Egg, scrambled	1	6	1.3	0.5
Egg white	1 oz (30 g)	3.6	0.8	0.34
Tuna, canned	4 oz (120 g)	22	3.8	1.7
Ground beef, 93% lean, cooked	4 oz (120 g)	24	4	1.8
Flank steak, cooked	4 oz (120 g)	31	5.3	2.4
Peanuts, roasted	1 oz (30 g)	8	1.1	0.5
Cottage cheese	1/2 cup	14	3.1	1.4
Yogurt, flavored, low-fat	6 oz (180 g)	7	2	0.8

induced muscle damage, improve recovery, support immune function, and assist in maintaining blood sugar levels.

BCAAs may also increase growth hormone (GH) circulation, which is responsible for promoting muscle growth and increasing strength. Of the three, leucine is the most heavily researched, and it appears to have the most influence on protein synthesis—that is, in the adult population. The use of BCAA supplements has not been studied in youth athletes.

BCAAs were being consumed long before the development of BCAA supplements; they are easy to get by eating an adequate amount of high-quality protein. Table 6.1 summarizes the BCAA content of popular foods. Not only is this a safe and reliable way for teens to get enough BCAAs, but also, these whole-food sources offer complete protein and other vitamins and mineral that they need.

Beta-Hydroxy-Beta-Methylbutyrate (HMB)

HMB, a product of the breakdown of the branched-chain amino acid leucine, is found naturally in foods such as catfish and grapefruit. Studies in adult athletes have shown that HMB may slow the breakdown of muscle and protein. Other potential benefits include increasing muscle mass, decreasing body fat, increasing anaerobic capacity, and (for those who are beginning a strength training program) boosting strength levels (Durkalec-Michalski and Jeszka, 2016; Wilson et al., 2013). There is very little research on the use of HMB in the adolescent population, although this seems to be a big area of interest for sport science researchers.

Because the beneficial role of HMB includes the promotion of muscle mass, only athletes at the appropriate developmental age (Tanner stage 4 or 5; see chapter 1) would likely benefit. There are two forms of HMB that have been used: calcium HMB (HMB-ca) and a free acid form of HMB (HMB-FA); HMB-Ca is the more popular form. One study examined the effects of 3 grams per day of calcium HMB (HMB-Ca) on elite male and female adolescent (13 to 18 years old, Tanner stage 4 or 5) volleyball players during the first seven weeks of their training season (Portal et al., 2011). The results showed that muscle mass increased and fat mass declined in the HMB-Ca group but not in the placebo group. In addition, upper- and lower-body strength improved. No changes in hormone status occurred with supplementation. Although this shows some promise for the use of HMB in adolescent athletes, no way do we have enough evidence to safely recommend this supplement to growing athletes. More evidence is needed before a dosing recommendation can be safely made.

Youth athletes can focus on dietary strategies to increase their HMB production, such as those recommended in chapter 3, although meeting the dosage recommendations used in research through food is not practical. According to the International Society of Sports Nutrition position stand on HMB, an athlete would need to eat more than 600 grams of high-quality protein to obtain the amount of leucine (60 g) necessary to produce the 3-gram daily dosage used in adult human studies (Wilson et al., 2013).

Glutamine

Glutamine is an amino acid found in skeletal muscle and blood. When the body is under stress, such as after heavy training or competition, glutamine is released into the bloodstream and acts as an important fuel source for immune system cells. Athletes supplement with glutamine to prevent or recover from an illness or injury. Although glutamine supplementation in the adult population is considered safe, the evidence to support its role in preventing illness, treating illness, or improving performance does not support the claims. Glutamine supplementation is not recommended for youth athletes. Instead, they should focus on making sure their sport fueling plan includes adequate protein, with sources spread out over the course of the day (see chapter 3 for examples).

Creatine

Creatine is made in the body from three different amino acids. Ninety-five percent of the body's creatine is stored in the muscle, where it gets turned into phosphocreatine. Phosphocreatine acts as an energy source, but it's only enough for a few seconds of action, such as during an extra muscle contraction. Creatine is also found naturally in some foods and can be purchased as a dietary supplement: creatine monohydrate.

Creatine itself does not produce bigger muscles; it allows the muscles to train harder. For example, an athlete using creatine may be able to finish one extra rep because the muscle is loaded with creatine. This harder training then leads to improved muscular strength, increased muscle mass, and, over time, improved athletic performance. In adults, creatine is one of the most widely researched and commonly used ergogenic aids. Its popularity likely comes from its suggestive benefits, which include increased muscle size, strength, and performance during short bouts of high-intensity exercise. Although past researchers questioned the safety of creatine, current evidence in the adult population suggests that it is safe.

Much less is known about the safety and efficacy of creatine supplementation in youth athletes. One study evaluating creatine supplementation in elite junior swimmers found that short-term supplementation may improve power output and swimming performance (Juhasz et al., 2009). Others studies in children and adolescents have evaluated its use relative to a variety of medical conditions (Balsom et al., 1994; Smith et al., 2014). Although no study has indicated harmful side effects in teenagers, we cannot say with certainly what the long-term effects might be. To date, very little is known about creatine supplementation in youth athletes.

The lack of evidence is surely not stopping youth athletes from experimenting. Surveys on supplement usage consistently list creatine as a top dietary supplement used by youth athletes. One survey of 1,349 high school football players showed that 30 percent had used creatine supplements (McGuine, Sullivan, and Bernhardt, 2001). I have worked with youth athletes who did not even realize they were taking creatine. That's because it is often added to protein and meal-replacement powders as well as mixed into the concoction of ingredients in other dietary supplements. This makes dosing, as well as safety and effectiveness, an issue. The long-term effects that creatine supplementation may have on youth athletes' growing bodies are unknown, especially if they begin use early and do not control how much they use. Could overuse from a young age negatively affect how the supplement could benefit them in the future? Is it safe for growing bodies? These are questions we cannot answer. Although the studies of creatine supplementation in growing children suggest that it appears to be safe, it is wise to focus on maximizing the training program and eating plan first. Dietary creatine is found in some animal products, and there are trace amounts in plant foods, but reaching the dosing amount used in research is unlikely with food. A mixed diet provides about 1 gram of creatine per day. See table 6.2 for creatine amounts in common food sources.

Table 6.2   Food Sources of Creatine

Food	Serving	Creatine (mg/serving)
Herring, raw	(3 oz, 90 g)	553-850
Pork, raw	(3 oz, 90 g)	425
Salmon, raw	(3 oz, 90 g)	383
Beef, raw	(3 oz, 90 g)	383
Cod, raw	(3 oz, 90 g)	255
Milk	(1 cup)	24

© Academy of Nutrition and Dietetics, *The health professional's guide to popular dietary supplements*, 3rd ed., 2007. Reprinted with permission.

Protein Powders

Should I just have a protein shake after my workout? If I had a dollar for every time I was asked that question, I would be rich. Protein powders are popular and appear to be safe—that is, if what the label says is in the package is true. These products fall under the same manufacturing guidelines as other dietary supplements. Protein powders are not necessary, but they may help youth athletes who are on the go and do not eat many animal products.

Protein powders are dietary supplements that contain a high percentage of protein. In addition to protein, many are fortified with other ingredients such as vitamins, minerals, greens, fat, and grains. The sources of protein in protein supplements include whey, casein, soy, hemp, rice, and pea. Many are sold as concentrates, isolates, and hydrolysates, but concentrates and isolates are the two most common. The main difference is that isolates have a slightly higher percentage of protein than concentrates do, because the nonprotein components have been removed. Both protein isolates and protein concentrates can be partially broken down, or hydrolyzed, resulting in slightly faster absorption. Protein isolates and protein hydrolysates are more expensive because of the increased concentration of protein.

Both whey and casein are derived from animal products and are therefore a complete source of protein. Soy, hemp, brown rice, and pea protein are plant based, and the protein content varies among the varieties. The type of protein powder chosen should be based on the athlete's goals and taste preferences.

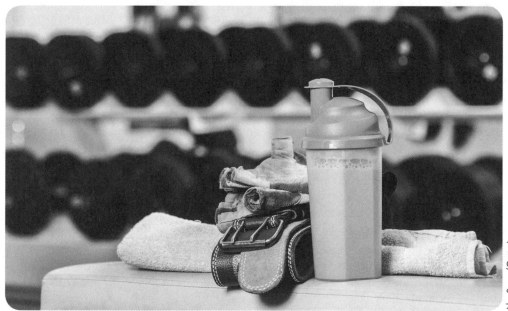

AlexSava/Getty Images

Protein shakes are a popular choice among young athletes, especially after exercise, but they are not all created equal. It is important to make sure that the protein or meal-replacement powder that you use after activity will support your performance goals.

All varieties have strengths and weaknesses. Table 6.3 lists popular types of protein supplements, their characteristics, and their food sources.

As discussed in chapter 3, the protein needs of a growing teenager depend on developmental age as well as individual goals and training intensity, duration, and timing. Most young athletes, even those with increased needs, are getting more than enough protein without having to rely on supplementation. Protein powders do provide an easy and portable way to reach protein needs, but relying on them too much can displace other valuable nutrients (see chapter 3). It is smart to get protein from foods rather than supplements. Whole-food protein sources provide other beneficial nutrients as well. Many protein foods are packed with zinc, iron, magnesium, calcium, omega-3 fatty acids, B vitamins, vitamin E, and vitamin D. Table 8.4 in chapter 8 is a comprehensive list of food sources of protein.

Table 6.3 Characteristics of Protein Powders

Type	Characteristics	Food sources
Whey	Derived from milk; complete protein; highly digestible, high concentration of BCAAs, including leucine; often recommended for postworkout recovery; dissolves well in water. Whey protein isolate is lactose free and therefore recommended for those with lactose intolerance.	Dairy products: milk, cheese, yogurt
Casein	Derived from milk; complete protein; absorbed slightly more slowly and steadily than whey; often recommended for meal replacements and before bed.	Dairy products: milk, cheese, yogurt
Soy	Derived from soy; plant-based complete protein source; less water soluble than whey; may have cardiovascular benefits.	Soybeans, soy nuts, soy milk, tofu, tempeh
Hemp	Plant based; lower protein content than other protein powders; contains essential fatty acids (omega-3); higher fat and carbohydrate content than other protein powders; hypoallergenic; higher in fiber, which slows digestion and absorption, which may have benefits in weight loss	Hemp drink (dairy alternative), hemp seeds, foods made with hemp (breads, crackers, etc.)
Brown rice	Plant based; hypoallergenic, gluten free, neutral taste; economical; higher carbohydrate content than other powders; source of B vitamins.	Rice (the concentration of protein is low)
Pea	Plant based: hypoallergenic; highly digestible; economical; may improve satiety, which may have benefits in weight loss.	Peas (the concentration of protein is low)

Meal-Replacement Powders and Weight Gainers

Meal-replacement powders (MRPs) often get clumped in with protein powders, but they are much more than that. In addition to providing high-quality protein, they usually include carbohydrate, fat, vitamins, minerals, and sometimes more. Although meal-replacement powders are touted as complete meals containing the perfect blend of nutrients, not all products fit that bill.

Meal-replacement powders vary significantly and are marketed for a variety of uses. Products marketed toward weight loss tend to be moderate in calories and are suggested to be used in place of a meal. However, youth athletes do not need meal replacements to control their weight. Other meal replacements are marketed to athletes wanting to gain weight. These products tend to be higher in calories, and the suggested use is between meals.

Although meal-replacement and weight-gainer powders should never replace a full meal, they do offer an easy and convenient way for youth athletes, especially those who are struggling to gain weight, to get calories on the go. However, be sure to check the Nutrition Facts label and ingredients list closely. Because many of these products are marketed to athletes looking to bulk up, they sometimes include other ergogenic ingredients such as creatine and stimulants.

Vitamins and Minerals

Vitamins and minerals are vital nutrients that play many roles in the body. They are largely involved in energy metabolism and digesting food and are often marketed to athletes suffering from fatigue. However, vitamins and minerals do not have calories and therefore do not supply energy. Their role in energy metabolism is to unlock the energy trapped inside carbohydrate, protein, and fat.

There is no benefit to consuming vitamins and minerals beyond the recommended dietary allowance (RDA), unless there is a known deficiency. Because teenage athletes tend to eat a lot of food, they should be able to meet their daily requirements without additional supplementation.

Chapter 3 addresses the importance of iron, calcium, and vitamin D. Although I chose to highlight only those three nutrients as a concern in athletes, a deficiency in any vitamin or mineral requires attention. An athlete with a dairy allergy, for example, may need to take a calcium supplement to meet the daily requirement for calcium. An athlete who follows a strict vegan diet because he has restricted the nutrients present in animal products such as vitamin B_{12} may need to take a vitamin B12 supplement. In the case of a known deficiency or insufficiency, a supplement may be necessary for bringing levels up to the normal range. Eating balanced meals and including nutrient-dense snacks between meals can help ensure proper nutrition.

Omega-3 Supplements

Recall from chapter 2 that omega-3 fatty acids are recommended as part of a healthy diet. Also recall that eating fatty fish a few times a week is the easiest way to reach this goal. The problem is that most Americans do not eat much fish. That's where supplements come in. The sale of omega-3 supplements has hit the sport nutrition industry in full force. This section tells you what you need to know.

Contrary to claims, the value of omega-3 fatty acids for athletic performance is mixed and inconclusive. A recent review of the literature concluded that although research is extensive, we cannot assume at present that omega-3 supplementation is effective in meeting the claims. Data are lacking to support its use in reducing the inflammatory response to exercise, delaying muscle soreness, or improving overall performance. There appears to be some promise in the use of omega-3 supplements for those who suffer from exercise-induced bronchoconstriction due to asthma. One study in youth wrestlers suggested that omega-3 supplementation during intensive wrestling training improved pulmonary function during and after exercise.

No DRI has been established for omega-3 fatty acids, but more is certainly not better. In fact, one of the concerns with using supplements over food is taking too much. The FDA recommends that consumers not exceed a daily total of 3 grams of EPA and DHA (two omega-3 fatty acids) from all sources and no more than 2 grams per day from a dietary supplement. Because omega-3 fatty acids can thin the blood, higher doses can increase the risk of bruising, especially in athletes, given their activities. Those who choose to supplement their diets with fish oil supplements should choose wisely. Remember, the FDA does not regulate supplements in the same way as drugs, so the amount listed on the label may be different from what you actually get. Also keep in mind that the recommendations for omega-3 fatty acids are for adults. Because no level or recommendation has been established for children or adolescents, I recommend that youth athletes focus on increasing their intake of omega-3 fatty acids through food sources, not dietary supplements.

Stimulants and Botanicals for Performance

Many of the following stimulants and botanicals are marketed for performance and are found in other dietary supplements (including energy drinks) and not necessarily as single supplements. Read labels carefully.

Caffeine

Caffeine is a stimulant found naturally in many foods and beverages. It is also added to many sport nutrition products and is a major component of energy drinks.

Most of the research on caffeine as an ergogenic aid has focused on endurance sports. Adult athletes use caffeine to improve endurance, delay fatigue, and enhance fat loss. Caffeine is often marketed as a fat burner; although there may be a slight increase in resting metabolic rate after ingesting caffeine, there is no evidence of a significant effect on fat loss or weight loss. The main benefit of caffeine appears to be its impact on the central nervous system, which makes exercise feel easier and reduces fatigue.

Caffeine affects people differently. Whereas one person may feel awake and alert, another may feel jittery and anxious. Because of its ergogenic effect, many companies have added caffeine to their products, but too much caffeine is counterproductive. Some unwanted side effects are anxiety, irritability, diarrhea, and insomnia. Caffeine also interferes with the absorption of certain vitamins and minerals, including iron and calcium, which are both of concern in youth athletes.

The use of caffeine as an ergogenic aid has not been studied in growing athletes. There is increased concern over the use of energy drinks in this population because many contain high levels of caffeine as well as herbal sources of caffeine (see the section Energy Drinks later in this chapter). Caffeine at those levels is not recommended, especially for young athletes who want to perform well. In addition to the previously mentioned negative side effects, there is the potential for caffeine intoxication, which could affect sleep. Remember, if sleep is cut short or disrupted, the body does not get the time it needs to complete all of the phases of muscle repair. The release of hormones that regulate growth and appetite also gets disrupted. The National Collegiate Athletic Association (NCAA) includes caffeine at high concentrations on its list of banned substances.

Guarana

Guarana is a central nervous system stimulant that is marketed for weight loss, to enhance athletic performance, and to reduce mental and physical fatigue. It is commonly found in energy drinks. It contains not only twice as much caffeine as coffee but also theophylline and theobromine, two chemicals that are similar to caffeine. There is no solid evidence that it improves athletic performance. It is not recommended for children or teenage athletes.

Because guarana contains caffeine, taking it with other herbs and supplements that contain caffeine can increase both the harmful and the helpful effects of caffeine. There is also some concern that combining caffeine, ephedra (an illegal and banned substance), and creatine might increase the risk of serious side effects. It is reported that too much caffeine may decrease creatine's beneficial effects on athletic performance.

Ginseng

Ginseng comes in many varieties, but the kind found in many popular energy drinks is referred to as Panax ginseng. It is used to improve thinking, concentration, memory, work efficiency, physical stamina, and athletic endurance. Although the claims persist, studies have shown that taking Panax ginseng for up to eight weeks does not improve athletic performance. It is deemed possibly safe when used in the short term, but researchers believe it may have hormone-like effects that could be harmful with prolonged use. The most common side effect is insomnia. Ginseng is not recommended for youth athletes.

Echinacea

Echinacea is a popular herbal supplement widely used to prevent and treat the common cold and other infections. The research on echinacea's effectiveness in treating the common cold is mixed. Some scientific evidence suggests that taking echinacea products when cold symptoms are first detected may reduce symptoms; other studies show no benefit. In one study conducted on healthy men, a modest dose of echinacea daily for 28 days improved breathing capacity during exercise (Whitehead, 2012). Taking echinacea along with caffeine might result in too much caffeine in the bloodstream and increase the risk of side effects. There is no evidence to support a benefit in youth athletes; therefore, it is not a recommended supplement.

L-Carnitine

L-carnitine is an amino acid that is naturally produced in the body. Its main job is to transport fatty acids into cells to be used as energy. L-carnitine is commonly included in the mix of substances added to energy drinks. Athletes use L-carnitine to burn fat during exercise or improve energy levels. Intense exercise has been linked to a decrease in L-carnitine blood levels, although research on the use of L-carnitine for improving athletic performance is inconsistent. Some studies in adults show that it may improve endurance performance; others do not. There are no studies to support the use of L-carnitine in youth athletes.

Ephedra

Ephedra (often labeled as ma huang) is an herb marketed for weight loss and athletic performance. In April 2004, the FDA banned the use of ephedra-containing products after growing increasingly aware of adverse effects. Side effects reported were headaches, increased heart rate, increased blood pressure, insomnia, and death. The dietary supplement industry challenged that ban, stating that no adverse effects were reported at low doses; a U.S. federal court later overturned the ruling, allowing low-dose ephedra-containing supplements to be sold in the United States. Concerns about the safety of these supplements are so serious that certain states have enacted their own bans; ephedra remains illegal to sell or purchase in those states. Ephedra is banned by the National Collegiate Athletic Association, International Olympic Committee, and National Football League. It is deemed unsafe for adults and children and has no place in the diets of young athletes.

Herbs, Spices, Phytonutrients, and Antioxidants

Long hours of training day after day can put a lot of strain on a youth athlete's body. This intense training causes an inflammatory response, which can negatively affect the immune system and ultimately result in decreased performance. The inflammatory reactions that occur in the body are complex. To break it down into terms youth athletes understand, I tell them this: If you are ill, injured, or inflamed, you will not perform at your best. If you want your body to work for you, you need to eat right.

One easy (and delicious) way to combat inflammation and support the immune system is to eat a diet that is high in antioxidants and anti-inflammatory foods. The following are a few that are being studied for their potential anti-inflammatory effects.

Ginger

Ginger is an herb. The stem, referred to as the rhizome, is used as a spice, a medicine to treat stomach issues, and a pain reliever for issues such as arthritis and muscle soreness. In the world of sports medicine and nutrition, the interest is in its potential anti-inflammatory properties. Some evidence suggests that ginger can reduce pain in adults suffering from osteoarthritis. It has also shown to reduce hip and knee pain related to arthritis. The results of studies comparing ginger with nonsteroidal anti-inflammatory drugs are mixed. Studies on the use of ginger for muscle pain are also contradictory.

No research shows that ginger helps reduce inflammation in youth athletes. Nevertheless, for athletes who are suffering from inflammation, incorporating a little ginger into the meal plan can't hurt, and it tastes good. It can easily be added to a smoothie or soups or baked into a batch of homemade energy bars.

Turmeric (Curcumin)

Turmeric is derived from the root of the turmeric plant. It contains curcumin, the yellow-colored active ingredient known for its antioxidant and anti-inflammatory properties. It is commonly used to flavor curry powders and other foods in Indian cooking. Turmeric found its way into the world of sports because of its potential as an anti-inflammatory agent. Although much of the research was conducted in animals, athletes are taking note. According to a report published in the American Botanical Council's publication *HerbalGram (2015)*, sales of herbal dietary supplements that contain turmeric, or curcumin, as the primary ingredient grew by 30.9% from 2013 to 2014.

Before you run out and purchase a turmeric, or curcumin, supplement, understand that much more evidence is needed, especially in human trials and adolescents. In the meantime, turmeric can easily be added to color and flavor foods. Try adding it to rice, scrambled eggs, or smoothies. It also tastes good mixed with lemon as a marinade for chicken, tossed with roasted vegetables, or added to soups.

Garlic

Garlic is an herb best known as a flavoring agent in food. Over the years, it's been touted as a way to prevent heart disease, cancer, osteoarthritis, colds, and fungus, among other conditions. Compounds extracted from garlic have been shown to exhibit anti-inflammatory properties. In the world of sport performance, garlic has been investigated for its influence on muscle soreness after exercise as well as on endurance. Two studies suggest a potential benefit of garlic in these areas.

When it comes to garlic, you either like it or you don't. If you wish to add it to your bucket of anti-inflammatory foods, you can easily add it to soups, stews, salad dressings, marinades, and dips. However, I do not recommend adding garlic to your next smoothie. You may never drink one again!

Tart Cherry Juice

Tart cherries and tart cherry juice are a hot topic these days not only in the sport literature but also among athletes. Cherries contain anthocyanins, compounds that block inflammation while helping to prevent muscle damage. Like ginger and turmeric, they are thought to provide a similar but natural alternative to nonsteroidal anti-inflammatory drugs for pain. There is evidence to support their antioxidant and anti-inflammatory properties, especially in adult endurance athletes. There are no studies available on the use of tart cherries or tart cherry juice in youth athletes.

Few companies today market tart cherry juice to athletes. To incorporate tart cherries into your diet, add them to a smoothie or drink tart cherry juice. Tart cherries can also be added to salads or yogurt or one of the homemade energy bar recipes in chapter 11.

These are only a few ways to boost your intake of antioxidants and anti-inflammatory foods. Many foods—blueberries, sweet potatoes, apples, green tea, kale, dark chocolate, and many others—offer a variety of flavonols that work in similar ways to fight in your body's defense. That is why eating a variety of foods each day is so important.

The amount of any herb, spice, or plant that is used in research studies will be difficult to obtain on a day-to-day basis, especially for busy youth athletes. Rather than stressing about how to meet your ginger needs for the day, for example, just look for ways to incorporate a variety of these foods into your meal plan. Add tart cherries to your next smoothie, put a pinch of turmeric into your scrambled eggs, then sauté chicken in garlic for dinner. Small incorporations of these ingredients will add up to a good dose of phytonutrients over the course of the day and contribute to your overall health.

Energy Drinks

The use of caffeine-containing energy drinks has drastically increased in the last few years, and much of that increase is due to marketing promoting their perceived ergogenic effects. Energy drinks are marketed as a quick and easy way to boost energy and mood. They often contain large amounts of caffeine and sugar along with other ingredients such as B vitamins, amino acids, and herbal stimulants (such as guarana and ginseng). They can contain up to 80 milligrams of caffeine per serving (the equivalent of a cup of coffee). Some brands have more. Caffeine, mixed with herbal compounds, can cause nervousness, irritability, increased heart rate, and insomnia. In a study of 90 athletes, some were given an energy drink 60 minutes before an exercise session, and others were given a placebo. The athletes who received the energy drink reported a greater prevalence of side effects such as insomnia, nervousness, and activeness when compared to the placebo group (Salinero et al., 2014). Although excess caffeine alone affects people differently, the mix of caffeine with other herbal ingredients can exacerbate the effects.

Energy drinks are very popular among youth athletes. Warnings on product labels stating that they are not recommended for children do not stop teens from drinking them. One popular energy drink company has sponsored athletes as young as 11. Companies tend to target young males with the endorsement of top athletes. Millions of teens have consumed energy drinks without any negative effects, but the Poison Control Center has expressed alarm over the use of these products, stating that the drinks may cause anxiety, dehydration, and, in rare cases, seizures and heart problems (Reissig, 2009). The FDA Center for Food Safety and Applied Nutrition (CFSAN) Adverse Event Reporting System (CAERS) collects reports of events and complaints from consumers. (2013). Consumers have reported symptoms such as hot flashes, anxiety, sleep disorders, hemorrhages, seizures, and death. In 2010, the cable channel ESPN brought huge attention to the issue when it reported on a 17-year-old high school football player who suffered a seizure after drinking two 16-ounce (480 ml) cans of an energy drink. The two cans contained a total of 520 milligrams of caffeine.

A huge concern with the overconsumption of energy drinks is the risk of heat-related illness, a potentially deadly concern in youth athletes (see chapter 3 for more on hydration). Ingesting a concoction of caffeine and herbs before beginning a training or practice session, especially in the heat, is a recipe for disaster.

Although many youth athletes report that they drink energy drinks to increase energy, they can actually zap energy. Because these products directly stimulate the central nervous system, athletes perceive that they have more energy, but the effects are short lived. In actuality, energy drinks can result in insomnia, which leaves an athlete feeling fatigued the next day. In an attempt to increase energy, another energy drink is consumed, and the cycle continues, as shown in figure 6.1. Anything that disrupts a solid sleep cycle can negatively affect performance. Youth athletes should not consume energy drinks.

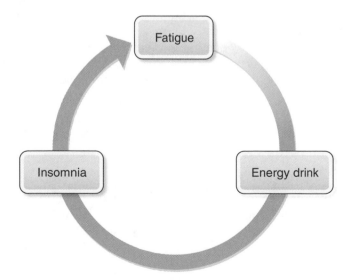

Figure 6.1   Effect of energy drinks on sleep.

Energy Drinks Versus Sport Drinks

There is still a lot of confusion about the difference between sport drinks and energy drinks. And be assured, there is a huge difference. Energy drinks often contain a higher concentration of carbohydrate (8 to 11 percent) than sport drinks (6 to 8 percent). This can delay gastric emptying (how slowly nutrients leave the stomach) and slow down the absorption in the gastrointestinal (GI) tract, especially if the beverage is consumed quickly. Sport drinks are designed to be rehydration beverages to consume during and after activity. They contain an appropriate level of electrolytes to promote maximal absorption of fluid by the GI tract.

Sport drinks are designed with athletes in mind. Energy drinks are not. Table 6.4 compares the two.

Table 6.4 Comparison of Energy Drinks and Sport Drinks

	Sport drink	**Energy drink**
Purpose	Replace fluid and electrolytes lost in sweat during and after activity.	Gain quick energy.
Carbohydrate	The 6% to 8% carbohydrate solution encourages the consumption of water to maintain normal hydration during exercise.	The 8% to 11% carbohydrate solution may delay gastric emptying and slow the absorption of nutrients in the GI tract. Not recommended for athletes.
Other ingredients	Electrolytes: Sodium, potassium. The sodium in sport drinks helps to replace sodium losses in sweat. It also stimulates thirst.	Stimulants such as caffeine, guarana, ginseng, or other herbs. May also include large doses of B vitamins. The mix of stimulants may result in negative and dangerous side effects that can interfere with sport performance.
Label	Nutrition Facts	Supplement Facts

In its "Position Statement and Recommendations for the Use of Energy Drinks by Young Athletes," the National Federation of State High School Associations (NFHS) Sports Medicine Advisory Committee (SMAC) strongly recommends the following (2014):

- Water and appropriate sports drinks should be used for rehydration as outlined in the NFHS "Position Statement and Recommendations for Maintaining Hydration to Optimize Performance and Minimize the Risk for Exertional Heat Illness."

- Energy drinks should not be used for hydration prior to, during, or after physical activity.
- Information about the absence of benefit and the presence of potential risk associated with energy drinks should be widely shared among all individuals who interact with young athletes.
- Athletes taking over the counter or prescription medications should not consume energy drinks without the approval of their physician.
- Energy Drinks ARE NOT sports drinks and should not be used by athletes in training or competition.

Reprinted, by permission, from National Federation of State High School Associations Sports Medicine Advisory Committee, 2014, Position statement and recommendations for the use of energy drinks by young athletes. [Online.] Available:www.nfhs.org/media/1014749/nfhs-smac-position-statement-for-use-of-energy-drinks-october-2014.pdf [June 14, 2016].

Energy Gels, Chews, Beans, and Blocks

Popular with endurance athletes, energy gels (or chews, blocks, or beans) are highly concentrated sources of energy sold in single-serve packages. They are a portable fuel source specifically for use during longer-duration activity. Some athletes find them beneficial as a quick source of carbohydrate on competition day, especially between events. Products vary by brand and type, but most contain a mixture of simple carbohydrate for quick digestion and absorption to provide immediate energy. They also contain electrolytes (sodium and potassium), although less than you would find in a sport drink. Several products on the market today include other ingredients, such as caffeine, herbal blends, B vitamins, and amino acids. You can even find a gel with ginger. What these concentrated energy sources do not have is water! If you try these products, make sure to drink sufficient water to process the carbohydrate and prevent dehydration. Read labels carefully before using these products.

Should Youth Athletes Use Dietary Supplements?

I read a tremendous amount of research on dietary supplements, ergogenic aids, and performance-enhancing products. As I've tried to point out throughout this chapter, most of the research is on adults, not children and adolescents. Although many parents and coaches are anxious to help their young athletes succeed, recommending dietary supplements is not the answer. Children and teenagers are not miniature adults. It is not clear how a child's body will tolerate or metabolize supplements, nor is it the time to experiment. In fact, that is why more research does not exist in that population. Exposing growing children and adolescents to dietary supplements for the purpose of testing is unethical and could disrupt their growth and development. As a nutrition scientist and a mom, I agree.

The National Federation of State High School Associations (NFHS) Sports Medicine Advisory Committee (SMAC) published a "Supplements Position Statement" on the topic (2014), which states the following:

> The NFHS Sports Medicine Advisory Committee (SMAC) strongly opposes the use of dietary supplements for the purpose of obtaining a competitive advantage. Research shows that there continues to be widespread use of dietary supplements by adolescent and high school athletes, despite considerable safety concerns. Dietary supplements are marketed as an easy way to enhance athletic performance, increase energy levels, lose weight, and feel better. Adolescents are more susceptible to peer pressure and these advertising messages, which may increase the incidence of dietary supplement usage and reinforce a culture more concerned about short-term performance rather than overall long-term athletic development and good health.

Reprinted by permission from NFHS Sports Medicine Advisory Committee, 2014.

Nevertheless, considering the wide range of products that fall under the umbrella of this term, some dietary supplements may be OK and even helpful. As you learned in chapter 3, certain vitamins and minerals are nutrients of concern in youth athletes. Supplementing the diet with these well-researched nutrients, such as vitamin D and iron, may help to avoid nutrient deficiencies. Protein powders may help athletes, especially vegan athletes or those who avoid animal products, meet their protein needs. Weight gainers may help athletes who have super-high caloric needs get the extra fuel for their performances. But before considering any dietary supplement, remember to do your homework. These questions can help:

- Is it safe for growing athletes?
- Is it proven effective for growing athletes?
- Is it contaminated?

Any respectable health care practitioner would want this proof before recommending a product to a growing child or adolescent athlete. Unfortunately, the evidence to support the safety and efficacy in this population is simply not available. Even in products that seem to be safe, the risk of contamination is real. Use one of the resources in the section Finding Reliable Information to answer the three questions. Use the information in this chapter to educate yourself on why your youth athlete may want a supplement, what the claims are, what the potential risks are, and what the current research shows.

Paul Klinger, business development executive at Informed-Choice, speaks from experience when he suggests being extra cautious of botanical (plant-based) ingredients that have higher concentrations of naturally occurring steroidal and stimulant agents. He also reminds athletes to steer clear of dietary

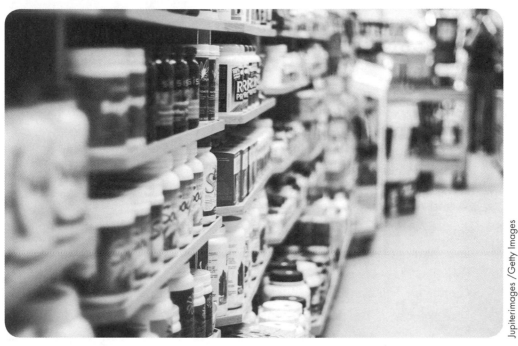

It is important that you receive information on dietary supplements from reliable sources. Most store clerks lack the education to properly guide consumers on safe supplementation.

supplements claiming to be testosterone boosters. As Klinger states, "Many products will say all-natural, which implies that it is safe" (personal communication). But if it really boosts testosterone, it likely has something in it that's potentially harmful. Remember that products labeled as fat burners and weight-loss promotors tend to have higher rates of stimulants and could contain steroidal compounds. Some preworkout formulas contain stimulants and botanicals that may be considered prohibited substances in sport or potentially dangerous to consumers. It is understandable that youth athletes want a competitive edge as they seek early entrance onto junior teams or college scholarships. But dietary supplements are not the quick-fix pills, potions, and powders they are made out to be.

Finding Reliable Information

To answer the preceding questions about supplements, you need to make sure your resources are legitimate. All too often, youth athletes get their advice from the wrong places. I recently asked high school athletes where they learn about dietary supplements; the answers included coaches, trainers, advertisements, health food store clerks, Internet sites, parents, and peers. Although some of these resources may be helpful, others are not. Most employees at supplement stores lack the education to properly guide consumers on the purchase of safe supplements.

Where to Find Reliable Information

The resources listed next are reliable sources that can help you make informed decisions.

Sport-Specific Agencies and Organizations

Drug Free Sport www.drugfreesport.com

Supplement Safety Now www.supplementsafetynow.com

TrueSport of the U.S. Anti-Doping Agency (USADA) www.usada.org/truesport

World Anti-Doping Agency www.wada-ama.org

Resources for Supplement Information

U.S. National Institutes of Health Office of Dietary Supplements http:ods.od.nih.gov

Center for Science in the Public Interest https://cspinet.org

Natural Medicines Comprehensive Database www.naturaldatabase.com

Supplements Watch www.supplementswatch.com

Organizations Addressing Supplement Purity

Informed-Choice www.informed-choice.org

- Tests supplements and ingredients on behalf of reputable manufacturers and suppliers, including banned substances.
- Tests every batch, verifying that there are no banned or prohibited substances.
- Tests multiple samples to assess the risk of cross-contamination from other products manufactured in the same facility.

NSF, Certified for Sport Program www.nsfsport.com

- Confirms that products do not contain any of the 180+ substances banned by major athletic associations.
- Verifies that the contents of the supplement actually match what is printed on the label.
- Verifies that there are no unsafe contaminants in the tested products.
- Verifies that the product is manufactured at a facility audited by NSF for quality and safety.

Banned Substances Control Group www.bscg.org

- Certified Drug Free Supplement Certification Program tests supplements to ensure that they are free of drugs that could lead to a positive drug test or cause harmful health effects.

- Testing menu aligns with the World Anti-Doping Agency prohibited list.
- Products tested by this group carry the BSCG Certified Drug Free seal.

Aegis Sciences Corporation www.aegislabs.com

- Independent anti-doping laboratory
- Provides a mobile app to quickly and easily identify the presence of banned substances in dietary supplements, based on the ingredients list.

U.S. Pharmacopeial Convention (USP) www.usp.org

- Offers third-party independent verification services for dietary supplement finished products and dietary ingredients.
- Products that meet the criteria for this program carry the USF Verified Mark symbol on the package.

No one organization or person will be able to answer all of your questions on dietary supplements. Do your homework. Make no assumptions on safety. Consider that the best option may be to avoid dietary supplements altogether. Sport dietitian Chris Rosenbloom, professor emerita of nutrition at Georgia State University, suggests smartphone apps that can help parents, coaches, and young athletes evaluate dietary supplements. Aegis Shield and NSF both have free apps. "I know that some will take supplements, so I encourage them to be informed rather than rely on Dr. Google," says Rosenbloom (personal communication).

Talking to Youth Athletes About Dietary Supplements

If you are a parent, coach, or trainer, and a young athlete asks you about dietary supplements and products to boost training efforts, don't disregard the question. Doing so is unlikely to result in their losing interest; instead, they will likely just go elsewhere (e.g., the Internet) for information. Just as we guide our teenagers to the best training facilities and encourage them to eat their vegetables, we need to educate them on the reality of dietary supplements, ergogenic aids, and other performance-enhancing drugs. Even if you are certain that your youth athlete is not taking them, there is a good chance he has heard of them and possibly even considered trying one. Some athletes, even after knowing the risks, will be tempted to try them.

When talking to youth athletes about supplements, remember these key points:

- Make the information relevant. Teenagers may not be interested in research study results or supplement statistics, but they will relate to the youth athletes who played their sport and suffered consequences. Share resources and stories, such as that of Taylor Hooton, a high school athlete who committed suicide as a result of abusing anabolic steroids.

- Keep an open mind about ergogenic aids and dietary supplements. If your athlete believes that you are totally against supplements, she may not even consider talking to you about them. Dismissing her means a missed opportunity to educate her and help her find proven ways to meet her goals.

- Share the NCAA list of banned substance with your athletes. This is a great way to approach the subject and educate them on what is ahead if they are interested in pursuing an athletic career at the collegiate or professional level. Be sure to point out that caffeine at high levels is on the list.

- If you are a parent, ask your child's coach or trainer his or her stance on dietary supplements right from the start. Ask questions and demand evidence of protocols or recommendations that you do not understand.

- Stay up to date on ergogenic aids and pay attention to which ones are being discussed among young athletes. Ask questions.

- Use your resources and teach youth athletes to use resources too! Download mobile apps such as Aegis Shield or NSF so that you have them at your fingertips.

Remember the discussion in chapter 1 on forming habits? Children learn a lot more than just eating and exercise habits from a young age; they also learn integrity, values, and morals from the adults and other role models around them. When the interest in dietary supplements becomes more important than the emphasis on hard work and eating right, sport training takes a turn for the worse. What starts off as an innocent recommendation can quickly lead to interest in other supplements and stimulants. Most youth athletes have not perfected their day-to-day diets enough to be considering supplementation. Parents, coaches, and trainers must be strong advocates for the sport nutrition practices that have been proven safe and effective, such as the ones outlined throughout this book.

If you want to help your youth athletes perform better and succeed over the long term, focus on a performance-enhancing diet and strategies that are proven to work, such as the following:

- Challenging training program
- Eating plan that supports sport training, promotes proper recovery, and keeps athletes healthy and strong
- Adequate sleep for growth and development
- Adequate hydration
- Vitamin or mineral supplements only when dietary inadequacies or deficiencies have been identified

What the Experts Are Saying

Other sport dietitians say these are the biggest mistakes they see high school athletes make regarding dietary supplements:

High school athletes rarely understand how the products work, just that their buddies are using them. In addition, students believe that supplements are regulated.

Roberta Anding, MS, RD/LD, CSSD,
director of sports nutrition at Texas Children's Hospital

They get their information from the wrong sources so they hear only the marketing pitch or anecdotes but not the real science. In addition, some young athletes are not physically mature and will not gain muscle mass until they go through puberty, but they still think supplements will help.

Chris Rosenbloom, PhD, RDN, CSSD,
professor emerita of nutrition at Georgia State University

High school athletes often take the advice from the supplement store staff, which often results in purchasing a product that is not formulated correctly. Other mistakes I see are that they do not discuss it with their parents before purchasing it, and they take more than the recommended dose on the label.

Tavis Piattoly, MS, RD,
cofounder and director of nutrition at My Sports Dietitian

I see high school athletes taking a supplement without first consulting a parent, doctor, coach, athletic trainer, or board-certified sport dietitian about the type, dosage, safety, and legality, which is a big mistake. There are too many supplements on the market, combined with a lack of research on those under 18, which can lead to students' taking supplements that are not safe or effective and may even cause life-threatening issues.

Kim Schwabenbauer, RD,
CSSD, founder of Fuel Your Passion

The biggest mistake is thinking that supplements alone can help performance, recovery, or changes in body composition. Creatine instead of lunch will not help muscles grow, or an energy shot instead of a snack will not improve stamina, speed, or strength during practices or workouts. We need our athletes to be "fuelies," opting for the food plate, not the supplement bottle, as the way to eat well, play on, and do their best.

Leslie Bonci, RD, CSSD,
owner of Active Eating Advice

The biggest mistake high school athletes make is thinking that dietary supplements are magic bullets that can instantaneously boost their performance or enhance their muscle mass. Also, many do not understand that, when it comes to dietary supplements, more can be dangerous.

Linda Samuels, RD, CSSD,
performance nutritionist, Training Table Sports Nutrition

- Consideration of safe supplements, such as sport drinks or meal replacements, when they are appropriate and align with the athlete's goals

As sport dietitian Tavis Piattoly, RD, points out, "Supplements are not a magic pill and will have very little to any performance benefit if caloric intake is not sufficient to match or exceed energy expenditure."

Chapter 7

Identifying and Dealing With Disordered Eating

Food likes and dislikes, texture issues, and game-day rituals—these are a few of the reasons youth athletes eat or do not eat certain foods. It is normal to be concerned and question whether these preferences are normal; what seems like a strange eating habit to one person may be perfectly normal and healthy to another. Then again, maybe not.

Not all bizarre eating habits fall under the category of disordered eating, and not all athletes who have disordered eating have a diagnosable eating disorder. Some athletes may just not like certain foods or feel better when they avoid certain foods. Some athletes may even change their diets or eliminate certain foods because they were told to do so or they read that it is better for their sport performance. These athletes may just need to learn how and why to eat better. Other youth athletes, however, may have disordered eating or an actual diagnosable eating disorder. Figuring out which is which can be harder than you think.

When I opened my sport nutrition practice, I had minimal experience working with clients suffering from eating disorders (ED). I was well educated on the topic from my formal training in graduate school, and I had some exposure during my first job as a dietitian, but I had little experience counseling people with eating disorders. I did not focus on identifying or treating disordered eating because I did not think that I needed to; my specialty was in sport nutrition and helping athletes eat to perform. It did not take me long to learn that I was mistaken. Disordered eating is very common among youth athletes—more common than you may imagine.

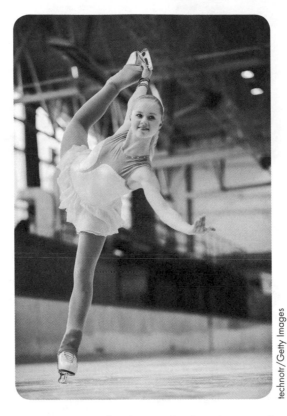

technotr/Getty Images

Eating disorders can occur in any sport, but they tend to be more prevalent in weight-class sports (sports where having a lower body weight enhances performance) and aesthetic sports such as gymnastics and figure skating.

Identifying Eating Disorders

Disordered eating in athletes often develops during adolescence. Remember from chapter 1 that this is a time of rapid body changes, especially for female athletes, and not all athletes are comfortable with their changing bodies. Coaches, trainers, and parents all play a critical role in helping youth athletes understand that their body changes are normal and necessary for healthy growth and development. They can also reinforce the importance of proper fueling. If there is a concern with body weight or composition, or if there is concern that an athlete is over- or underweight, a referral to the right professional is the best approach. Even coaches and parents who have the best intentions can say the wrong things about losing or gaining weight and set an athlete up for disordered eating. I know this because I see a lot of youth athletes with disordered eating in my practice.

As I set out to become an expert in the area, I was very interested in whether a higher incidence of eating disorders occurs in youth athletes than in non-athletes—and if so, why. Is it the culture? Are athletes more focused on body image? Or do the qualities that make a star athlete (i.e., being focused, highly motivated, coachable, and driven) make them susceptible to developing eating disorders? Many young athletes are hesitant to admit body image or weight fears, so they keep them to themselves. When I work with young athletes, it can take weeks before they admit to food fears. Youth athletes may also use sport to rationalize and justify their eating behaviors. In some sports, disordered eating is so common that it is viewed as acceptable.

Studies using questionnaires have found that high school athletes do not have a greater risk of developing eating disorders than their age-matched controls, although experts still question the results. Are disordered eating and eating disorders something that can be identified with a simple questionnaire? Many researchers believe that a clinical interview of the youth athlete, in addition to a questionnaire, is necessary to determine whether an athlete is at risk or if an eating disorder exists. One study that included clinical interviews revealed a higher prevalence of eating disorders among elite adolescent athletes than among controls (Martinsen and Sundgot-Borgen, 2013) supporting that theory. That evidence further supports the need for high schools to develop a protocol for screening for disordered eating and eating disorders in youth athletes, including face-to-face discussions. In an ideal world, all high schools would have a sport dietitian on the team who could do these screenings. And all athletic associations would be prepared to identify and help youth athletes struggling with eating or body image issues.

Even with tools in place, a sport dietitian is often the first practitioner to suspect an eating issue in an athlete. That makes sense because they see athletes who are having weight, health, and performance issues and those who are recovering from injury. Unfortunately, athletes who have disordered eating or eating disorders often end up with one of those consequences.

I have always considered myself a good counselor; I have a natural ability to read people and have always had good instincts. Although early in my career I lacked the professional experience and training to treat clients with eating disorders, I was good at detecting them. And my clients trusted me enough to share their concerns about food and body image. However, I was not an expert. When I suspected disordered eating or an eating disorder, I referred my client to a dietitian who specialized in that area. I was making referrals regularly, and it was heartbreaking. I could not believe how common disordered eating is among youth athletes. I realized that it did not feel right to work hard to develop relationships with every one of my clients, and when they finally trusted me enough to open up about their eating fears, I would send them to another dietitian for counseling. I was the expert who understood their sports and sport nutrition. I was also the expert they trusted to talk about their eating and body image fears. I wanted to help them improve their eating patterns. My athletes needed an expert in both sport nutrition and disordered eating. I decided it was time to dive into more training.

I attended conferences, interviewed colleagues who specialized in eating disorders, spoke with athletes recovering from eating disorders, and read study after study on the manifestations of disordered eating in athletes. I discovered that there are a variety of approaches to treatment. One thing is for sure: It takes a team of trained experts to help a youth athlete overcome an eating disorder. Coaches, trainers, and parents can educate themselves on the topic to help prevent disordered eating, but once it turns into something serious, athletes need expert help. Not only their sport careers depend on it; their health and well-being depend on it as well.

Types of Eating Disorders

In May 2013, the American Psychiatric Association published the *Diagnostic and Statistical Manual of Mental Disorders, Fifth Edition* (*DSM-5*). The *DSM* describes the specific criteria for diagnosing and classifying eating disorders. The three primary eating disorders with concrete diagnosable criteria are anorexia nervosa (AN), bulimia nervosa (BN), and binge eating disorder (BED). A fourth type, referred to as other specified feeding or eating disorder (OSFED), is characterized as disruptions in eating behavior that do not fall into the categories of anorexia, bulimia, or binge eating disorder. Although OSFED does not have specific criteria, it is just as serious. It is also the most common type of eating disorder.

Eating disorders appear to be issues about food, but they go much deeper than that. To date, no defined cause has been established, but several factors may affect their development. For one, there may be a genetic factor. Eating disorders often run in families and it is thought that the risk of developing an eating disorder may be determined by genetics. Social factors such as the pressure to obtain the ideal body may also play a role. Psychological factors or other mental health disorders such as depression, anxiety, obsessive-compulsive disorder, and low self-esteem can also contribute to the risk of developing an eating disorder. And interpersonal factors, such as a history of abuse, being bullied about body weight, traumatic life events, and simply having a difficult time expressing feeling, also come into play. It is not the job of a coach, trainer, or parent to diagnose an eating disorder. However, being familiar with them, their warning signs, and the potential health consequences can help them determine whether consulting an expert could help an athlete.

Anorexia Nervosa (AN)

Anorexia nervosa is characterized by a distorted body image, intense fear of being fat, and self-starvation that leads to severe weight loss. Following are the warning signs of anorexia nervosa:

- Dramatic weight loss
- Distorted body image; frequent comments about being fat or feeling fat

- Intense fear of gaining weight
- Preoccupation with weight, calories, fat grams, and food in general
- Feelings of guilt after eating
- High levels of anxiety, depression, or both
- Withdrawal from friends and activities
- Excuses for not eating, denial of hunger, and avoidance of mealtimes
- Strict food rules or rituals
- Abuse of laxatives, diet pills, or diuretics
- Excessive and compulsive exercise

Eating Disorders in Male Athletes

There is no doubt that males can develop eating disorders. It is a huge misconception that eating disorders are a female issue, and that belief can leave boys confused about whether their eating issues and body image concerns even classify as problems. It can also leave them feeling ashamed and attempting to hide their disorders. One study found that young men's belief that eating disorders affect only females led them to recognize their own symptoms of eating disorders only when they had become advanced (MacLean et al., 2015). Even today, the media portrays eating disorders as atypical of men. Eating disorders do not discriminate; pay attention to youth male athletes as well as females.

Eating disorders in males are similar to those in females, but they differ in terms of features. The age of onset tends to be later in males than in females. Males tend to be more concerned with body composition, especially building muscle and having a lean, muscular physique. They are also more likely to have been overweight before their eating disorder or to have been teased about their weight or size. Participation in weight-oriented sports such as wrestling, horse jockeying, and football can be a contributing factor. But disordered eating in youth male athletes is not limited to these sports. I have worked with male athletes dealing with disordered eating in a variety of sports, including hockey, rowing, baseball, wrestling, swimming, and dance. When I see male clients, it is rarely for an eating disorder; the complaint is often a decline in performance, a body fat percentage that has dropped below healthy guidelines, or the discovery that they are using unhealthy products to improve their physique. Most often, it is not until I work with the athlete and have built a trusting relationship that food issues emerge.

Bulimia Nervosa (BN)

Bulimia nervosa is characterized as bingeing (consuming a large amount of food) and then purging (getting rid of food). Symptoms include repeated episodes of bingeing and purging with the feeling of being out of control during a binge, inappropriate compensatory behaviors after a binge (such as the use of laxatives or diuretics, obsessive or compulsive exercise, or fasting), and extreme concern with body weight and shape. Following are the warning signs of bulimia nervosa:

- Evidence of bingeing (e.g., large amounts of food disappearing in a short time)
- Eating in private or hoarding food; hiding empty wrappers in unusual places
- Evidence of purging such as frequent trips to the bathroom after meals; signs of vomiting (hearing or smelling)
- Preoccupation with food
- Weight fluctuations
- Calluses on the backs of hands and knuckles from self-induced vomiting
- Excessive and rigid exercise regimens; comments regarding the need to burn off calories
- Abuse of laxatives, diet pills, or diuretics
- Discoloration or staining of teeth
- Broken blood vessels in the eyes or face from vomiting
- Complaints of, or admittance to, sore throat, heartburn, or reflux
- Feelings of shame and guilt resulting in anxiety, depression, or both
- Self-criticism and low self-esteem

Binge Eating Disorder (BED)

Binge eating disorder (BED) is characterized as repeated episodes of eating large amounts of food in a short time while feeling out of control during the eating episodes. Following are the warning signs of binge eating disorder:

- Eating large quantities of food, without purging behaviors, when not hungry
- Sense of being out of control when eating
- Eating until uncomfortably full
- Weight gain or obesity
- Feelings of shame and guilt or being disgusted by the behavior
- Eating alone; secretive eating or hiding food
- High levels of anxiety, depression, or both

Other Specified Feeding or Eating Disorder (OSFED)

Other specified feeding or eating disorder (OSFED) is a feeding or eating disorder that causes significant distress or impairment but does not fall into the category of anorexia, bulimia, or binge eating disorder. Warning signs and potential health consequences of OSFED are similar to, and just as severe as, those for the other eating disorders but less specific. Following are examples of the ways OSFED differs from the other three diagnosable eating disorders:

- All criteria are met for the diagnosis of anorexia nervosa, except that body weight is normal or above the normal range.
- All criteria are met for bulimia nervosa, except that the binge eating and other compensatory behaviors occur at a lower frequency.
- All criteria are met for binge eating disorder, except that binge eating occurs, on average, less than once a week or for less than three months, or both.
- Purging without bingeing (sometimes referred to as purging disorder).
- Night eating syndrome (NES), which is an ongoing, persistent pattern of late-night binge eating. Consuming large quantities of food occurs after the evening meal or after awakening from sleep, or both.

Other Forms of Disordered Eating

The previously listed eating disorders are the most recognized and most common, but many more have to do with body image concerns and unhealthy eating habits. Body dysmorphic disorder and muscle dysmorphia are forms of eating disorders that are seen in both girls and boys. Avoidant and restrictive food intake disorder and compulsive exercise are two more. The purpose of this chapter is not to overwhelm you with the criteria for every form of disordered eating but rather to open your eyes to the countless ways it can present. That said, there is one more type of disordered pattern I want to expand on.

Orthorexia nervosa (ON) starts as an innocent attempt to improve eating habits, but it can turn into an unhealthy fixation in some at-risk people. Those with orthorexia spend just as much time thinking about food as those with anorexia or bulimia, but rather than obsess about the calories, they think about the quality and purity of the food including how it was prepared, processed, and stored. This condition often starts very innocently. An athlete may change his eating habits for a good reason—for example, after learning that too much sugar can contribute to inflammation or that trans fat might raise LDL cholesterol. Learning something negative about a food or food group, whether it is true or not, can trigger orthorexia. In today's culture, fear sells; media outlets and trendy diet books use sensational words such as *dangerous, deadly,* and *toxic* to garner attention. These words fallen on the wrong ears can have devastating effects, especially on young athletes. Family habits, nutrition trends, or recent illnesses can also trigger orthorexia. The person often removes a food group or an ingredient initially (e.g., artificial sweeteners and colors, processed foods,

Allison

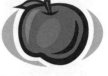

Allison was a 16-year-old starting tennis player who trained five or six times per week. She was 5 feet 2 inches (157 cm) tall and weighed 93 pounds (42 kg). When Allison decided to follow a vegetarian diet, her mom initiated a consultation to make sure it was providing adequate nutrition. Her mom was concerned because, since Allison had started to follow the diet, she had lost weight and her athletic performance had declined. Her usual body weight was 110 pounds (50 kg), meaning that she had lost 17 pounds (7.7 kg) in the past four months.

During the initial appointment, Allison and I discussed her eating habits, weight history, and weekly training regimen. I also learned that she had not menstruated in four months. Based on her symptoms, it was obvious that Allison was underfueling. But why?

I was curious about why Allison had chosen to follow a vegetarian diet, so we spent some time discussing that. Allison explained that her health teacher had showed the movie *Food, Inc.* during health class. After watching the movie and having a discussion about the ways animals are treated, Allison decided to become vegetarian. She also eliminated sugar after being told that it was toxic and bad for her body.

Allison had been given one-sided nutrition information that affected her decisions on what to eat and distorted her idea of what was healthy. She was not afraid of eating too many calories; she simply wanted to eat only healthy foods. Allison showed signs of orthorexia. Unlike many people who have orthorexia, Allison had removed everything she believed was unhealthy all at once. This left her following a low-calorie, low-nutrient diet that resulted in rapid weight loss, menstrual dysfunction, malnutrition, and poor performance. Her weight loss was not intentional; it happened because she had eliminated so many foods that she was left with hardly anything to nourish her body.

It took a few weeks, but Allison eventually started to acknowledge her food fears. She denied any fear of weight gain, but she admitted to being afraid to eat certain "unhealthy" foods and to avoiding certain social situations. She was lonely.

I created a plan that provided 100 percent of her nutrition needs but used only foods that she viewed as safe. The safe plan provided enough calories, carbohydrate, and nutrients to help her return to a healthy weight, start menstruating, and improve her performance while she was working through the psychological issues with her therapist.

fat, sugar, GMOs, processed foods). Over time, more foods and ingredients are removed, and the drive to be healthier and the fixation on eating only safe foods turn obsessive.

Bringing awareness to orthorexia is a personal passion, so much so that I write and speak on the topic regularly. Orthorexia can best be understood as healthy eating that is taken too far and becomes an excessive preoccupation (i.e., perfect eating). The term was first coined by Dr. Steven Bratman in 1997 and has gained recognition in recent years. At present, orthorexia is not a formal eating disorder, but more clinical reports are being published as it becomes more familiar to health care professionals. Validated diagnostic criteria have not been developed but have been proposed (Bratman and Dunn, 2016).

Orthorexia can be difficult to detect because those with the condition tend to be proud of, not embarrassed about, the way they eat. In extreme cases, the obsessive-compulsive behaviors become pathological and begin to dominate athletes' lives. They may withdraw from the team and avoid eating out because they do not trust others to prepare their food. Although they secretly want to spend less time thinking about food, as the obsession with healthy eating advances, so does their social isolation.

There is a difference between healthy eating and orthorexia. Just because a youth athlete eats healthy and takes pride in preparing her meals does not mean she has orthorexia. We encourage youth athletes to take time and consider what they put in their bodies, and we want them to eat healthy food. It is OK to strive for a great diet, but it should not get in the way of having a happy life. Table 7.1 shows a comparison to clarify the difference between healthy eating and orthorexia.

Because youth athletes with orthorexia do not necessarily restrict calories or the macronutrients required for good performance, athletic performance may not be affected initially. But over time, performance declines. Suffering from orthorexia can leave a young athlete feeling socially isolated, lonely, and anxious. Orthorexia left untreated can transform into anorexia.

Those who struggle with disordered eating do not always have behaviors that fit perfectly into one of the categories. It is not uncommon to shift among food restrictions, food elimination, bingeing, purging, and clean eating, and then back to food restrictions. What these disordered eating patterns have in common is an obsession with food and a disordered sense of what constitutes healthy eating.

My mission to become more educated in how disordered eating in athletes begins included interviews with athletes in recovery. Many female athletes recalled a comment by a coach that losing a few pounds would improve her performance. Although likely innocent, a comment such as that may be all that is needed to send a highly competitive athlete down the road to disordered eating. Coaches may not realize the influence they have over youth athletes, but let me tell you, it is powerful. Youth athletes look up to their coaches, and they are more

Table 7.1 Healthy Eating Versus Orthorexia

Healthy eating habits	Orthorexia
May limit processed foods and artificial ingredients or limit intake of saturated fat, trans fat, sugar, and sodium.	Completely avoids any foods viewed as unhealthy (which varies from person to person) to the point of having difficulty finding enough food to meet nutritional needs.
May try different diets or experiment with different diet choices such as eating vegetarian, going gluten free, or "clean eating."	Spends excessive amount of time thinking about what foods to eat.
Chooses to eat healthy items when eating out.	Avoids foods that are bought or prepared by others.
Plans meals ahead of time.	Spends hours prepping food and has anxiety over getting meals ready.
Usually skips dessert.	Never has dessert, even on special occasions.
Intends to make healthy choices but still socializes and enjoys life.	Becomes withdrawn and avoids social situations; suffers decreased quality of life.
Reads ingredients lists.	Obsesses over the ingredients in food.
Might feel bad about eating something viewed as unhealthy.	Ends eating episodes with a postmeal evaluation: satisfaction or guilt.

Female Athlete Triad

A major issue of concern in female athletes is a spectrum disorder referred to as the female athlete triad. It involves three components: low energy availability (with or without disordered eating), menstrual dysfunction, and low bone density.

Physically active females often present with one or more of the three components. Constant underfueling results in low energy, which can have significant effects on health and sport performance. This is especially true when disordered eating is present. A missed menstrual period might seem like a minor issue, but it is a signal from the body that something is wrong. Left untreated, menstrual abnormalities can progress to more serious complications, including amenorrhea and the medical conditions associated with that disorder. Low energy also has negative effects on bone density. Bone stress fractures are reportedly more common in females with menstrual irregularities or low bone mineral density (or both) and lead to the more chronic condition known as osteoporosis. An injured athlete cannot be the best athlete.

Although female athletes with disordered eating are at increased risk of developing the triad, not all athletes with low energy have eating disorders. Because the nutrition needs of growing adolescents are high, some athletes struggle to meet their nutrition requirements. Time constraints, lack of food availability, and lack of proper nutrition knowledge can all affect how much food an athlete eats. The most important thing to remember is that this is a serious issue. When low energy is identified and corrected in enough time, the progression to more serious complications (e.g., a clinical eating disorder, amenorrhea, osteoporosis) can be prevented. This requires screening, education, and open dialogues about the importance of eating right for growth, development, and sport performance.

The International Olympic Committee (IOC) went one step further when outlining the risks associated with the female athlete triad and low energy by introducing the term *relative energy deficiency in sport (RED-S)*. This expands on the three main components of the triad and acknowledges the complexity of the condition. It also recognizes that male athletes may be affected. Specifically, it highlights the other health consequences of relative energy expenditure in sport, including the impact it can have on growth and development (see figure 7.1).

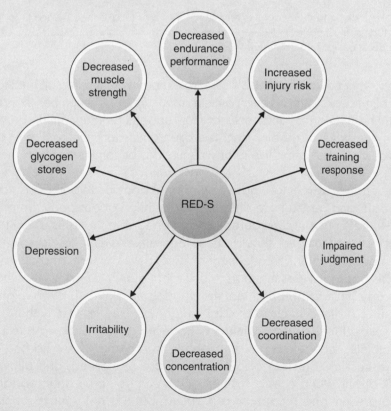

Figure 7.1 Potential effects of energy deficiency.
Reprinted from M. Mountjoy, J. Sundgot-Borgen, L. Burke, et al., 2014, "The IOC consensus statement: Beyond the Female Athlete Triad—Relative Energy Deficiency in Sport (RED-S)," *British Journal of Sports Medicine* 48:491-497, by permission of M. Mountjoy. Adapted from N.W. Constantini, 2002, Medical concerns of the dancer. XXVII FIMS World Congress of Sports Medicine, Budapest, Hungary, by permission of the author.

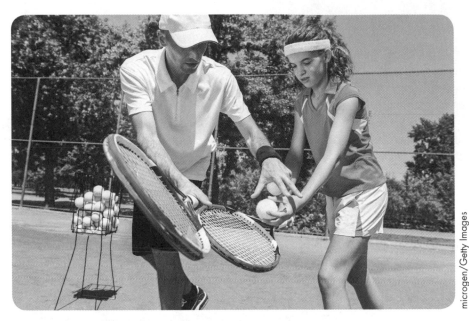

microgen/Getty Images

Young athletes look up to their coaches and are more likely to take their advice than that of other role models. It is important to keep the conversation on health and sport performance and not on body composition or weight loss.

likely to take their advice than that of other role models in their lives. It is critical to use caution when speaking to a young athlete about weight. Remember that prepubescent weight gain is normal and necessary for supporting an upcoming growth spurt. Athletes at this stage of development are often uncomfortable with their changing bodies and can be very sensitive to any discussions or comments about them.

Recommending weight loss based on normal body development is completely inappropriate and bad advice. In fact, any mention about body weight is risky business. To help prevent disordered eating or negative thoughts about food, parents, coaches, and trainers should encourage athletes to follow a sport nutrition plan that meets their nutrition needs for growth, development, and athletic performance. This book provides the tools to build that plan, no matter what the goal. If it has already been established that the developing athlete is overweight, follow the guidelines outlined in chapter 4 for weight loss and fat loss without dieting.

If you suspect that a youth athlete is not eating right and want to discuss it with the athlete, schedule a private meeting in a place where no one else can hear the discussion. Be clear about why you are concerned, and allow the athlete to talk openly. As a coach, trainer, or parent, you play an important role in helping to prevent and recognize a problem, but it is not your responsibility to be a therapist. Eating disorders require professional help. Once a problem has been identified, creating a treatment team, including a therapist, a dietitian, and a doctor, should be the priority. You can show the athlete that you care by taking an active role in identifying a treatment team and supporting that team.

Part III

Customize Your Sport Nutrition Plan

Chapter 8

Creating Your Personal Plan

When I begin working with a new athlete, the parents and athlete are eager for me to give them a meal plan that lays out exactly what to eat. But that is not what I do. Instead, I teach them how to create a meal plan for themselves. In this chapter, I am going to teach that to you!

Teenagers have enormous variances in nutritional needs. Recall our discussion on this topic from chapter 3: nutrition needs are influenced by not only the athlete's height, weight, and developmental age but also the sport, sport position, level of training, and goals. However, even with all of those things figured out, there is more to consider. A sport nutrition plan is no good if it doesn't work with the athlete's day-to-day schedule. Here are questions to consider when creating a personal nutrition plan:

- What is the athlete's training schedule?
- What is the athlete's school schedule?
- Are there individual and family barriers such as being able to afford food or having access to food?
- What are the athlete's food preferences?

If I handed you a predetermined meal plan, would you be able to follow it? Would it include foods you like? Would you understand how to swap one type of food for another, or would you eat the same thing every day just to stick to the plan? In my experience, the reason meal plans don't work (and diets too for that matter) is that people tend to follow the parts of the plan they like and ignore the parts they don't. The result is shortfalls in nutrition.

Rather than provide meal plans, I create what I refer to as individualized meal skeletons for my clients. I then use the skeleton to teach them how to plan meals. This chapter shows you how to create your own meal skeleton using the information provided in the first few chapters. This way, you can create your own meal plans based on your unique needs, food preferences, and training schedule.

Although planning meals may seem like a lot of work, it is one of the best skills a high school athlete can learn. You will learn not only how to eat to meet your current goals but also how to adjust your eating plan as your training and goals change. You can then carry this knowledge with you through your collegiate career, professional career, and life.

Have a pencil and paper ready because in this chapter I'll walk you step by step through the following process.

1. *Categorize foods.* You will learn which foods are considered carbohydrate, protein, and fat sources.

2. *Learn serving sizes.* You will learn how much of each food makes up a single serving.

3. *Estimate your nutrient needs.* You will use the information from the first few chapters to calculate your nutrition needs and determine how many servings of each macronutrient you need.

4. *Create a meal skeleton.* You will learn how to spread out the calories and macronutrients you need so that you eat the right amount of food at the right time.

5. *Create a meal plan.* Using the food charts, you will plug the foods you like into your meal skeleton.

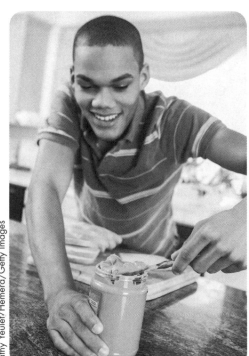

In addition, this chapter provides sample breakfast, lunch, dinner, and mini-meal choices. Recipes for many of the foods in the meal plans are in chapters 10 and 11. Many of the people I work with ask me for ideas and recipes, and they want to know exactly how they fit into the meal plan. This book does the work for you. Even though one-on-one nutrition counseling may be necessary at times, this book is meant to be the next best thing. Now, let's get started.

Learning to plan and prepare from a young age gives high school athletes an advantage. It is a skill that they will carry with them through their entire lives.

Cathy Yeulet/Hemera/Getty Images

Step 1: Categorize Foods

In early chapters you learned why you need to incorporate each of the macro-nutrients (carbohydrate, protein, and fat) into your meal plan. Now, you need to make sure you understand which foods fit into each category. I can tell you that most youth athletes—as well as their parents—are surprised to find out which foods are considered sources of carbohydrate. Learning how to categorize foods is the first step to building a meal plan that will properly support growth, development, and sport performance.

Which Foods Are Carbohydrate Sources?

Recall that carbohydrate is divided into complex and simple. In terms of the U.S. government icon MyPlate discussed in chapter 2, all five areas of the plate can provide carbohydrate, although some offer more choices than others. Choices from the grain, fruit, and vegetable sections all have carbohydrate. Milk and yogurt, which fall under the dairy group, are also sources of carbohydrate. From the protein section of the plate, we get carbohydrate from beans and legumes. Foods with added sugar also have carbohydrate. These foods, such as the sugar in a sport drink or candy, may not have a place on the My-Plate icon, but they are foods that youth athletes may consume on occasion. As you learned, some of the engineered sport foods have added sugar on purpose to provide the energy needed for long-distance or high-intensity activity.

Which Foods Are Protein Sources?

Remember that protein contains amino acids, which are used to build and repair body tissues. Protein occurs in most animal-based products such as red meat, poultry, fish, milk, eggs, and cheese as well as some plant-based foods such as soy, beans, and legumes.

Some foods are categorized as containing only protein (e.g., egg whites and boneless, skinless chicken breast that is very lean). Foods considered sources of both protein and fat include chicken thighs and whole eggs. Some foods are categorized as containing both protein and carbohydrate (e.g., beans and legumes).

The protein foods you choose should depend on your needs, goals, and training. You can choose foods that are either complete or incomplete proteins, but most, if not all, of your meals and mini-meals should include a source of protein.

Which Foods Are Fat Sources?

Dietary fat is an important fuel source for youth athletes. In chapter 2 you learned that dietary fat can be categorized as unsaturated fat, saturated fat, or trans fat. Many foods contain naturally occurring fat; many of the protein sources just mentioned fall into that category. Other foods have added fat (e.g., buttery crackers or a slice of birthday cake). Some foods have no or very little carbohydrate or protein and are considered fat sources only. These include oils, butter, nut butters, nuts, seeds, and salad dressings. When filling in your meal skeleton, make sure that all of your fat sources, both naturally occurring fats and all added fats, are included within your total fat servings.

Table 8.1 provides a quick glimpse into how to categorize foods. Remember that many carbohydrate sources are made with fat and fall under both categories, and many protein foods have naturally occurring fat and fall under both categories. Step 2 provides more specific information, including how much food makes up a single serving. From there, you will be able to determine how much food, or what your individual portion of food, should be.

Table 8.1 Food Categories

Carbohydrate	Protein	Fat
Starch (breads and cereals)	Beef	All oils
Starchy vegetables including beans and legumes	Poultry	Avocado
Fruit	Fish and shellfish	Butter and margarine
Nonstarchy vegetables	Eggs	Nuts
Milk and yogurt	Milk and yogurt	Seeds
Added sugar	Beans and legumes	Peanut and other nut butters
	Soy-based foods such as tofu and tempeh	Olives
	Cheese	

Step 2: Learn Serving Sizes

Now that you know how to categorize foods, you need to understand how much food counts as a single serving. Specific foods are not good or bad; it is how much of them you eat that affects your ability to attain your goals. For example, a piece of toast with peanut butter is a good choice before practice. It is a good way to top off glycogen stores while supplying a small amount of fat to prevent hunger. Change that portion size to three pieces of toast with gobs of peanut butter, and you will likely end up with a stomachache. Athletes, especially growing athletes, are unique in terms of the amount of food they need at one time. While one athlete may need to eat three servings of carbohydrate per meal, another athlete may need six servings. Knowing what counts as a single serving from each group is necessary for you to properly complete your meal skeleton.

A serving size is based on the number of grams of carbohydrate, protein, and fat in the food. The serving size is not necessarily the amount of food you will eat at one time; it is used only as a way to fill in your meal skeleton. A younger athlete may need two servings of carbohydrate at a breakfast meal, whereas an older athlete may need five servings. Table 8.2 shows you the number of calories and grams estimated to be in each nutrient to help you determine a single serving size. We talk more about that in step 4.

Table 8.2　Estimated Calories and Grams Per Serving of Each Nutrient

Nutrient	Grams per serving	Calories per serving
Carbohydrate	15	80
Protein	7	40
Fat	5	45

Carbohydrate Servings and Categories

Table 8.3 lists the serving size as well as the carbohydrate (CHO) and fat (FAT) count to use when adding those foods to your meal plan. Remember that some carbohydrate foods have fat in them.

Note that foods that are made with added sugar, such as candy, frozen yogurt, sugar-sweetened cereals, and sugary beverages, are also considered carbohydrate foods. They fall in the category of other sugars. Other foods, such as cakes, cookies, doughnuts, and ice cream, have added sugar and also added fat. There is no way I could list all of these foods in this book. The easiest way to determine how many servings these added sugars and fats make up is to look at the food labels. Remember that one serving of fat is equal to 5 grams. So, if an ice cream label indicates that 1/2 cup has 15 grams of fat, you can count your 1/2 cup of ice cream as three fat servings. If that same ice cream also has 15 grams of carbohydrate, you also count it as one carbohydrate serving.

Protein Servings and Categories

Table 8.4 is a list of protein foods with serving sizes and the nutrient count (PRO, CHO, FAT) to use when adding them to your meal plan. Remember that many protein foods have fat in them, and some have carbohydrate.

Dietary Fat Servings and Categories

The foods in table 8.5 are categorized as only fat. The list does not include the natural fat found in protein foods or the added fat in other foods. The amount of food has been adjusted so that they all provide 5 grams of fat, or 1 serving.

Table 8.3 Carbohydrate Food List

Starchy foods		
Food	**Serving size**	**Count as**
Bagel, mini (2 1/2 in., or 6.4 cm, diameter)	1	1 CHO
Bagel, small (3 in., or 7.6 cm, diameter)	1	2 CHO
Bagel, large (4 in., or 10 cm, diameter)	1	4 CHO
Bagel, thin	1	2 CHO
Bread	1 slice (1 oz, or 30 g)	1 CHO
Bun, hot dog or hamburger	1	2 CHO
Cereal, puffed	1 1/2 cups	1 CHO
Cereal, ready to eat, sweetened	1/2 cup	1 CHO
Cereal, ready to eat, unsweetened	3/4 cup	1 CHO
Corn, cooked	1/2 cup	1 CHO
Dinner roll, large	1 (2 oz, or 60 g)	2 CHO
Dinner roll, small	1 (1 oz, or 30 g)	1 CHO
English muffin	1	2 CHO
Granola	1/4 cup	1 CHO + 1 FAT
Hot cereal	1/2 cup, cooked	1 CHO
Naan bread	1 piece	3 CHO
Pancake, small (music CD size)	1	1 CHO
Pasta, cooked	1/3 cup	1 CHO
Peas, cooked	1/2 cup	1 CHO
Pita bread, large	1/2	2 CHO
Potato, baked, mini, red skinned	3	1 CHO
Potato, baked, with skin	3 oz, or 90 g	1 CHO
Potato, mashed	1/2 cup	1 CHO
Potato, oven baked (French fries)	12-15 French fries	1 CHO
Quinoa, cooked	1/3 cup	1 CHO
Rice cakes (4 in., or 10 cm, diameter)	2	1 CHO
Rice, cooked	1/3 cup	1 CHO
Squash, butternut	1 cup	1 CHO
Sweet potato (2 1/2 in., or 6.4 cm, diameter, 5 in., or 12.7 cm, long)	1	2 CHO

Starchy foods *(continued)*		
Food	**Serving size**	**Count as**
Tabbouleh (tabouli), prepared	1/2 cup	1 CHO
Taco shells, hard	2	1 CHO
Tortilla, flour (10 in., or 25 cm)	1	3 CHO
Tortilla, flour (6 in., or 15.2 cm)	1	1 CHO
Waffle, frozen	1	1 CHO
Starchy snacks		
Food	**Serving size**	**Count as**
Chips, baked	3/4 oz, or 21 g (13-18 chips)	1 CHO + 1 FAT
Chips, potato (regular)	1 oz, or 30 g (12-16 chips)	1 CHO + 2 FAT
Chips, tortilla	1 oz, or 30 g (8-13 chips)	1 CHO + 1 FAT
Cracker, Goldfish type	45	1 CHO + 1 FAT
Cracker, Cheez-It type	15	1 CHO + 1 FAT
Crackers, graham (2 1/2 in., or 6.4 cm, square)	3	1 CHO
Crackers, round butter type	6	1 CHO + 1 FAT
Crackers, saltine type	6	1 CHO
Popcorn, buttered	3 cups	1 CHO + 3 FAT
Popcorn, plain	3 cups	1 CHO
Potato, baked, mini, red skinned	3	1 CHO
Pretzels	3/4 oz, or 21 g	1 CHO
Rice cakes (4 in., or 10 cm, diameter)	2	1 CHO
Vanilla wafers, regular	5	1 CHO
Nonstarchy vegetables		
Food	**Serving size**	**Count as**
Most cooked vegetables	1/2 cup	1 CHO
Most raw vegetables	3 cups	1 CHO
Lettuce	No limit	FREE
Dark green leafy vegetables	No limit	FREE
Salsa, fresh	3/4 cup	1 CHO
Marinara sauce	3/4 cup	1 CHO

(continued)

Table 8.3 Carbohydrate Food List *(continued)*

Carbohydrate foods with plant-based protein		
Food	**Serving size**	**Count as**
Beans, baked	1/2 cup	2 CHO + 1 PRO
Beans, cooked (black, garbanzo, kidney, lima, navy, pinto, white)	1/2 cup	1 CHO + 1 PRO
Lentils, cooked	1/2 cup	1 CHO + 1 PRO
Fruit		
Food	**Serving size**	**Count as**
Apple, small	1 (4 oz, or 120 g)	1 CHO
Applesauce, unsweetened	1/2 cup	1 CHO
Banana, extra small	1 (4 oz, or 120 g)	1 CHO
Blackberries	3/4 cup	1 CHO
Blueberries	3/4 cup	1 CHO
Cantaloupe, cubed	1 cup (11 oz, or 330 g)	1 CHO
Grapefruit	1/2	1 CHO
Grapes	12	1 CHO
Honeydew melon, cubed	1 cup (10 oz, or 300 g)	1 CHO
Kiwi	1	1 CHO
Mandarin oranges, canned	3/4 cup	1 CHO
Mango	1/2 (5 1/2 oz, or 165 g)	1 CHO
Nectarine, medium	1	1 CHO
Orange, medium	1	1 CHO
Peach, medium	1	1 CHO
Peaches, canned	1/2 cup	1 CHO
Pear, medium	1/2	1 CHO
Pears, canned	1/2 cup	1 CHO
Pineapple, canned	1/2 cup	1 CHO
Pineapple, fresh	3/4 cup	1 CHO
Plums, fresh, small	2	1 CHO
Raspberries	1 cup	1 CHO
Strawberries, medium	15	1 CHO
Cherries, sweet	12	1 CHO
Tangerines, small	2	1 CHO
Watermelon, cubed	1 1/4 cups (13 1/2 oz, or 405 g)	1 CHO

Fruit juice

Food	Serving size	Count as
Apple juice	1/2 cup	1 CHO
Cranberry juice	1/2 cup	1 CHO
Grape juice	1/3 cup	1 CHO
Grapefruit juice	1/2 cup	1 CHO
Orange juice	1/2 cup	1 CHO
Pineapple juice	1/2 cup	1 CHO
Prune juice	1/3 cup	1 CHO

Dried fruit

Food	Serving size	Count as
Apples	3 rings	1 CHO
Apricots	9 halves	1 CHO
Blueberries	2 tbsp (30 g)	1 CHO
Cranberries	2 tbsp (30 g)	1 CHO
Dates	3	1 CHO
Figs	3	1 CHO
Prunes	3	1 CHO
Raisins, seedless	2 tbsp (30 g)	1 CHO

Milk, yogurt, and milk alternatives

Food	Serving size	Count as
Milk, fat free or low fat, 1%	1 cup	1 CHO + 1 PRO
Milk, 2%	1 cup	1 CHO + 1 PRO + 1 FAT
Milk, whole	1 cup	1 CHO + 1 PRO + 2 FAT
Milk, chocolate, fat free	1 cup	2 CHO +1 PRO
Milk, chocolate, whole	1 cup	2 CHO +1 PRO + 2 FAT
Soy milk, light	1 cup	1 CHO + 0.5 FAT
Soy milk, regular, plain	1 cup	1 CHO + 1 FAT
Almond milk, original	1 cup	0.5 CHO + 0.5 FAT
Almond milk, flavored	1 cup	1 CHO + 0.5 FAT
Almond milk, unsweetened, original or flavored	1 cup	0.5 FAT
Rice drink, flavored	1 cup	2 CHO
Rice drink, plain	1 cup	1 CHO

(continued)

Table 8.3 Carbohydrate Food List *(continued)*

Milk, yogurt, and milk alternatives *(continued)*		
Food	**Serving size**	**Count as**
Yogurt, Greek, plain, nonfat	5.3 oz (1 individual container)	0.5 CHO + 2 PRO
Yogurt, Greek, flavored, nonfat	5.3 oz (160 g, 1 container)	1 CHO + 2 PRO
Yogurt, plain, low fat	6 oz (180 g)	1 CHO + 1 PRO
Yogurt, fruit-flavored	6 oz (180 g)	2 CHO + 1 PRO
Yogurt, made with artificial sweetener	6 oz (180 g)	1 CHO + 1 PRO

Foods with added sugar		
Food	**Serving size**	**Count as**
Sport drink	20 oz (600 ml)	2 CHO
Sport gel	1	2 CHO
Sport beans	~16	2 CHO
Energy chews and blocks	~ 3	2 CHO

Sources: 1) US Department of Agriculture, Agricultural Research Service, Nutrient Data Laboratory. USDA National Nutrient Database for Standard Reference; 2) Academy of Nutrition and Dietetics, American Diabetes Association, 2014, *Choose your foods: Food lists for weight management.*

Table 8.4 Protein Food List

Lean protein		
Food	**Serving size**	**Count as**
Bacon, Canadian	1 slice	1 PRO
Beans and legumes	1/2 cup	1 CHO + 1 PRO
Beef jerky	3/4 oz	1 PRO +1 FAT
Chicken and turkey, boneless, skinless, white meat	1 oz (30 g)	1 PRO
Cottage cheese	1/4 cup	1 PRO
Deli meat: turkey, baked ham, chicken	1 oz (30 g)	1 PRO
Edamame	1/2 cup	1 CHO + 1 PRO
Egg whites	2	1 PRO
Shellfish	1 oz (30 g)	1 PRO
Tuna, canned in water	1 oz (30 g)	1 PRO
Fish, white	1 oz (30 g)	1 PRO

Protein with naturally occurring fat		
Food	**Serving size**	**Count as**
Chicken and turkey, skinless, dark meat	2 oz (60 g)	2 PRO + 1 FAT
Bacon, Canadian	1 slice	1 PRO
Bacon, pork based	2 slices	1 PRO + 2 FAT
Bacon, turkey	2 slices	1 PRO + 1 FAT
Beef patty, from a restaurant	4 oz (120 g)	4 PRO + 4 FAT
Beef, ground, 85% lean	2 oz (60 g)	2 PRO + 2 FAT
Beef, ground ,93% lean	2 oz (60 g)	2 PRO + 1 FAT
Beef, trimmed of visible fat, prime cuts of beef	2 oz (60 g)	2 PRO + 2 FAT
Cheese, American, Colby, cheddar, Swiss, provolone	1 oz (30 g)	1 PRO + 2 FAT
Cheese, feta, mozzarella	1 oz (30 g)	1 PRO + 1 FAT
Cheese, reduced fat	1 oz (30 g)	1 PRO + 1 FAT
Egg	1	1 PRO + 1 FAT
Hot dog, average size	1	1 PRO + 2.5 FAT
Hot dog, light (pork, turkey, beef)	1	1 PRO + 2 FAT
Pork, loin	2 oz (60 g)	2 PRO + 1 FAT
Deli meats, high fat: bologna, pastrami, hard salami, pepperoni	4 slices	1 PRO + 2 FAT
Sausage, turkey	2 links	1 PRO + 2 FAT
Tuna, in oil	1 oz (30 grams)	1 PRO + 0.5 FAT
Tofu	1/2 cup	1 PRO + 1 FAT

Sources: 1) US Department of Agriculture, Agricultural Research Service, Nutrient Data Laboratory. USDA National Nutrient Database for Standard Reference; 2) Academy of Nutrition and Dietetics, American Diabetes Association, 2014, *Choose your foods: Food lists for weight management.*

Table 8.5 Dietary Fat Food List

Food	Serving size	Counts as
Avocado	2 tbsp (30 g)	1 FAT
Butter and margarine	1 tsp (5 g)	1 FAT
Butter and margarine, light	1 tbsp (5 g)	1 FAT
Cream cheese	1 tsp (5 g)	1 FAT
Cream cheese, low fat	2 tbsp (30 g)	1 FAT
Half and half	2 tbsp (30 ml)	1 FAT
Mayonnaise	1 tsp (5 g)	1 FAT
Mayonnaise, light	1 tbsp (15 g)	1 FAT
Oil	1 tsp (5 ml)	1 FAT
Olives, large	10	1 FAT
Salad dressing	1 tbsp (15 ml)	1 FAT
Salad dressing, light	2 tbsp (30 ml)	1 FAT
Sour cream	2 tbsp (30 g)	1 FAT
Peanut butter	2 tsp (10 g)	1 FAT
Nut butter	2 tsp (10 g)	1 FAT
Almonds	8	1 FAT
Macadamia nuts	3	1 FAT
Peanuts	10	1 FAT
Pistachios	16	1 FAT
Pecans	5 halves	1 FAT
Walnuts	5 halves	1 FAT
Chia seeds	1 1/2 tbsp (23 g)	1 FAT
Flaxseeds	1 tbsp (15 g)	1 FAT
Hemp seeds	1 tbsp (15 g)	1 FAT
Pumpkin seeds	1 tbsp (15 g)	1 FAT
Sunflower seeds	1 tbsp (15 g)	1 FAT

Sources: 1) US Department of Agriculture, Agricultural Research Service, Nutrient Data Laboratory. USDA National Nutrient Database for Standard Reference; 2) Academy of Nutrition and Dietetics, American Diabetes Association, 2014, *Choose your foods: Food lists for weight management.*

Step 3: Estimate Your Nutrient Needs

Now that you know how much food makes up a single serving of carbohydrate, protein, and fat, the next thing you need to know is how many servings you need to be eating. As mentioned earlier, serving sizes do not change; however, the number of servings consumed varies from athlete to athlete. To create an individualized meal plan for yourself, you need to know how many servings of carbohydrate, protein, and fat you need to reach your goals. To do that, you need to calculate your daily needs. This next section walks you through calculating your nutrition needs based on your specific requirements.

What Are Your Caloric Needs?

Calculating the caloric needs of children and adolescents is much more difficult than calculating those of adults. Recall the discussion in chapter 3 of the challenge of figuring out the physical activity levels (PAL) for youth. In my practice, I use table 8.6 as a first step in determining overall energy needs. Most youth

Table 8.6 Determining PAL for Youth

Start your calculation of energy needs here . . .	. . . if you . . .	Examples
Sedentary PAL[1]	Do not participate in any sports, exercise, or activity.	Athletes suffering an injury or taking time off from sport
Low active PAL[2]	Are a recreational athlete with 1-hour practice times 1 to 3 times per week with a 1-hour game on the weekend.	• Athletes participating in beginner sport teams, such as the local township or YMCA baseball, soccer, or basketball team • Athletes participating in recreational cheerleading or gymnastics, or taking dancing or gymnastics lessons
Active PAL[3]	Spend ~1 hour a day being active or participating in moderate-intensity training for your sport.	• Athletes who participate in beginner sports and also train or practice on their own ~1 hour most days of the week • Athletes who participate in sports that are lower impact or more skill based, such as golf, baseball, and diving
Very active PAL[4]	Spend over 1 hour per day participating in activity.	Competitive athletes who practice or train more than 1 hour per day, especially those participating in higher-intensity activity.

[1]Sedentary PAL = rare in children
[2]Low active PAL = less than 1 hour/day of activity
[3]Active PAL = Approximately 1 hour/day of activity
[4]Very active PAL = More than 1 hour/day of activity
Adapted from J. Otten, J.P. Hellwig, and L.D. Meyers for Institute of Medicine of the National Academies, 2014, *Dietary Reference Intakes: The essential guide to nutrient requirements* (Washington, DC: National Academies Press), 84.

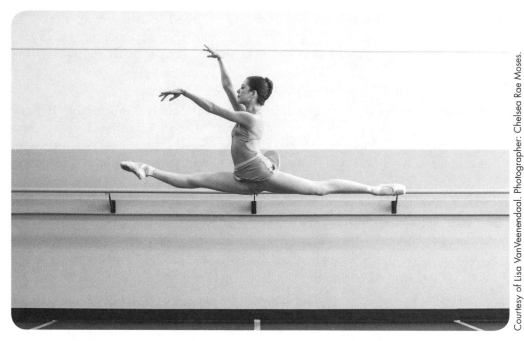

Courtesy of Lisa VanVeenendaal. Photographer: Chelsea Rae Moses.

Calculating the daily nutrition needs of a young athlete is not as easy as adding up numbers. Even within the same sport, some days are high-calorie-burning days while others are low-calorie-burning days.

athletes in competitive sports fall under the active PAL[3] or very active PAL[4] category, although some are in the lower categories. Remember, this is an estimate; adjustments may be necessary based on individual goals, body composition, developmental age, and intensity of training.

The examples in table 8.6 are intended to be a guide. Some sports have days when the training intensity is very high and other days when it is much lower. Cheerleading is a good example. Cheerleading is a high-calorie-burning activity when the athletes are practicing the dance part of the routine, but a lower-calorie-burning sport when they are working on stunts, which is more skill work. Gymnastics is a high-calorie-burning sport on a day when tumbling is the focus, but a lower-calorie-burning sport when working on skills, such as on the balance beam. Some athletes, such as high school swimmers, practice two or more hours per day. Athletes with that level of training will most likely have caloric needs even higher than what is listed on the chart. Remember that the meal skeleton and meal plan are meant to support your performance goals. If your goals include changes to body composition, such as gaining weight or decreasing body fat, additional adjustments may be needed (see chapter 4 for guidance).

What Are Your Protcin Needs?

Recall from chapter 3 that your protein needs will vary based on the type of activity you do as well as your goals. Use figure 8.1 to calculate your estimated protein needs.

Figure 8.1   Calculating My Protein Needs

	Lower range of protein needs	Higher range of protein needs	Record your range
If you participate in an endurance sport	Your weight in kg* × 1.2 = _____	Your weight in kg × 1.4 = _____	
If you participate in a strength sport	Your weight in kg × 1.2 = _____	Your weight in kg × 1.7 = _____	

*To convert your weight from pounds to kilograms, divide your weight in pounds by 2.2: Your weight in pounds (lb) _____ ÷ 2.2 = _____ your weight in kilograms (kg).

From H.R. Mangieri, 2017, *Fueling young athletes* (Champaign, IL: Human Kinetics).

Some youth athletes participate in strength and endurance activities evenly. Do not let that confuse you. If you are not sure whether to follow the recommendations for endurance or strength, calculate both. Remember, most athletes are already eating more protein than they need in a day but may not be eating it at the right time. Your meal skeleton will help you evenly distribute your intake so that you get the most out of your consumption.

Keep your protein range handy so you can record it later in figure 8.5, My Daily Nutrient Needs.

What Are Your Carbohydrate Needs?

Calculating carbohydrate needs in youth athletes is not easy. Just as with total energy, the amount of carbohydrate required depends on your age, sex, and body weight as well as the intensity of your activity, total daily energy expenditure, and sport. Figure 8.2 is a general guideline to help you calculate your carbohydrate needs.

Keep your carbohydrate range handy so you can record it later in figure 8.5, My Daily Nutrient Needs.

Figure 8.2   Calculating My Carbohydrate Needs

Intensity of activity	Carbohydrate needs (grams per kilogram of body weight per day)	Calculate your needs (lower range)*	Calculate your needs (higher range)*
Light training	3-5	Your weight in kg** _____ × 3 = _____	Your weight in kg _____ × 5 = _____
Moderate training	5-6	Your weight in kg _____ × 5 = _____	Your weight in kg _____ × 6 = _____
Heavy training	7-8	Your weight in kg _____ × 7 = _____	Your weight in kg _____ × 8 = _____

*Younger athletes should eat at the lower levels; older adolescent males will likely fall closer to the higher levels.

** To convert your weight from pounds to kilograms, divide your weight in pounds by 2.2: Your weight in pounds (lb) _____ ÷ 2.2 = _____ your weight in kilograms (kg).

From H.R. Mangieri, 2017, *Fueling young athletes* (Champaign, IL: Human Kinetics).

What Are Your Dietary Fat Needs?

When you determine daily nutrition needs, fat is the last nutrient to be calculated, but that it is not because it is not important. In fact, as you learned in chapter 3, fat is a valuable fuel source for youth athletes. Dietary fat has more calories per gram than carbohydrate or protein. Once you have calculated the amount of carbohydrate you need to fuel your brain and working muscles and the protein you need to build and repair muscles, the calories that are left will come from fat. To figure this out, you have to first calculate how many calories you have already determined you need from carbohydrate and protein. Figure 8.3 shows how to calculate the dietary fat needs for a very active 68-kilogram (150 lb) 16-year-old male; use figure 8.4 to calculate your own needs.

Figure 8.3 Calculating My Dietary Fat Needs

	Your daily grams	Grams per nutrient	Calories from nutrients	Total calories
Step 1: Record your total estimated calorie needs.				**3,663**
Step 2: Determine your total calories from carbohydrate: grams of CHO/day × Calories per gram of CHO	**68** kg × **8** g/kg = **544**	Total grams (544) × calories/ gram (4)= 2,176	**2,176**	
Step 3: Determine your total calories from protein: grams of protein/day × Calories per gram of protein	**68** kg × **1.6** g/kg = **109**	Total grams (109) × calories/ gram (4) = 436	**436**	
Step 4: Add your calories from carbohydrate and protein (steps 2 and 3).			**2,176+436**	**2,612**
Step 5: Subtract the number in step 4 from total calories (step 1). This is your total calories from **fat**.			**3,663– 2,612**	**1,051**
Step 6: Divide the calorie amount in step 5 by the calories per gram of fat (**9**). This gives you the grams of fat you need for the day.	**117**	**9**	**1,051**	

Check yourself! The percentage of your calories from fat should be 25 to 35 percent of your total calories. To check, divide your calories from fat into your total calories. Using the example from figure 8.3, it looks like this:

$$1,051 \div 3,663 = 29\% \text{ of total calories from fat}$$

If the calories from fat exceeds 35 percent of your total calories, you may have underestimated how much carbohydrate you need. Remember, the calorie level that you selected from the EER table (table 3.1) should match the activity level you choose from the carbohydrate needs chart (figure 8.2). Most youth athletes will not have daily fat needs that exceed 30 percent of their total calories. Older adolescent athletes who have really high calorie needs or difficulty gaining weight may be closer to 35 percent of total calories from fat. Try to choose the majority of your fat from healthy sources, such as nuts, seeds, olive oil, and omega-3 fatty acids found in fatty fish.

Now it's your turn to calculate your fat needs. When you're finished, keep your number handy so you can record it later in figure 8.5, My Daily Nutrient Needs.

Figure 8.4 Calculating My Dietary Fat Needs

	Your daily grams	Calories per gram	Calories from nutrients	Total
Step 1: Record your total estimated calorie needs.				
Step 2: Determine your total calories from carbohydrate.		**4**		
Step 3: Determine your total calories from protein.		**4**		
Step 4: Add your calories from carbohydrate and protein (steps 2 and 3).				
Step 5: Subtract the number in step 4 from your total calories (step 1). This is your total calories from **fat**.				
Divide the calorie amount in step 5 by the calories per gram of fat (**9**). This gives you the grams of fat you need for the day.		**9**		

From H.R. Mangieri, 2017, *Fueling young athletes* (Champaign, IL: Human Kinetics).

Now you have everything you need to determine how many servings of each nutrient you should eat each day. If you have not already filled in figure 8.5, My Daily Nutrient Needs, do that now. Both the total grams and total calories columns can be filled in.

Once you have the total calories from each nutrient and the grams per nutrient recorded in figure 8.5, you can estimate how many servings of each nutrient that you will need. To determine this, divide the total calories of each nutrient (carbohydrate, protein, and fat) by the number of calories estimated in each serving. (Recall from table 8.2.)

Remember that creating a meal skeleton is not an exact science. While I am sharing with you a lot of information about calories, calories per gram, and calories per serving, this program is not meant for you to count calories. It is meant for you to estimate how many servings of food you need to make it easy for you to create a meal plan.

If you attempt to calculate these numbers precisely and try to have them add up to 100 percent, you will likely be unsuccessful and become very frustrated. Keep in mind that the total calories in each serving of food will vary based on the specific brand as well as any other nutrients in the food. For example, half a cup of cereal is considered one serving of carbohydrate. That means that it is estimated to have about 15 grams of carbohydrate and 80 calories. However, depending on the brand that you eat, your cereal choices may have 17 grams of carbohydrate and 90 calories. That is all right. It is still considered to be one serving because it is close to the 15 grams and close to the 80 calories. Remember, these are estimates. The important thing is that your meal skeleton include a balance of macronutrients and micronutrients over the course of the day, not that your calorie amount be precise.

Using the same very active 68-kilogram (150 lb) male from earlier figures, I will show you how to calculate your servings per day (see figure 8.6). Then, in figure 8.7, it is your turn to calculate your own daily servings of carbohydrate, protein, and fat.

Figure 8.5   My Daily Nutrient Needs

	Grams	Calories
Total daily calories		
Daily carbohydrate		
Daily protein		
Daily fat		

From H.R. Mangieri, 2017, *Fueling young athletes* (Champaign, IL: Human Kinetics).

Figure 8.6 Calculating Daily Servings of Each Nutrient for a Very Active 16-Year-Old Male

Nutrient	Total daily calories/nutrient	. . . divided by	Total servings per day
Carbohydrate	2,176	80	**27**
Protein	436	40	**11**
Fat	1,051	45	**23**

Figure 8.7 Calculating My Daily Servings of Each Nutrient

Nutrient	Total daily calories/nutrient	. . . divided by	Total servings per day
Carbohydrate		80	
Protein		40	
Fat		45	

From H.R. Mangieri, 2017, *Fueling young athletes* (Champaign, IL: Human Kinetics).

Step 4: Create a Meal Skeleton

A meal skeleton is an outline of how much food you need to eat at one time and when to eat it. It is the foundation of the meal plan. In step 3 you calculated how many servings of each macronutrient (carbohydrate, protein, and fat) you need for the day, but there is much more to it. As a growing athlete, you need the vitamins and minerals those macronutrients provide to meet your health and performance goals. To ensure you are meeting your nutrition needs, it is important to choose a variety of foods, especially when it comes to carbohydrate. By choosing all of your carbohydrate servings from one group (e.g., starch), you will miss the key vitamins and minerals present in fruits, vegetables, and dairy products. In this section you will learn how to spread your total daily carbohydrate calories over many food sources. Remember, the meal skeleton helps you balance your total daily servings of food into meals and mini-meals. Answer the following questions to help you build a meal skeleton that is best for you and your schedule:

How many meals are you currently eating?

The number of meals is important because your first sport nutrition plan should not be very different from your current eating plan. When I work with clients, I strongly consider how they are eating before we get started. Trying to get an athlete who eats only two meals a day to eat eight meals a day is not realistic. This chapter will help you create a near-perfect nutrition plan, but that does not do you much good if you can't or won't follow it. When you create your plan, be realistic about what you can do. As you get better and feel better, you can come back to this chapter and create a new meal skeleton.

Nutrient Overview

Throughout this book, you have been learning about nutrients and the importance of eating a variety of foods and distributing those foods over the course of the day. Let's review some of the key points here.

Carbohydrate

- Choose a variety of carbohydrate sources from all of the food groups.
- Aim for at least five servings of fruits and vegetables a day.
- Aim for three servings of dairy a day.
- Include complex carbohydrates, especially those with fiber, in your meal plan.
- Avoid high-fiber foods immediately before activity.
- Limit added sugar and simple sugar to times around activity.

Protein

- Choose a protein source with each meal or mini-meal (snack). The exceptions are directly before activity or during activity.
- Keep protein evenly distributed by getting 20 to 30 grams (three or four servings) of protein at each meal and 10 to 15 grams (one or two servings) at each mini-meal (snack).

Fat

- Have a fat source at each meal or mini-meal. Sometimes it will be in your carbohydrate or protein selection.
- Limit fat intake immediately before activity, and avoid fat during activity.
- Try to evenly distribute your fat servings throughout the day. Eating too much fat at one time will cause you to be too full, resulting in your not wanting to eat your next meal or mini-meal. As a rule, try to limit fat to no more than 25 grams (five servings) per meal.

Vitamins and Minerals

- Review the charts in chapter 2 that show you how to meet your daily needs for essential vitamins and minerals. Be sure to include some of those foods in your meal plan.
- Remember, a variety of foods means a variety of nutrients.

How intense are your training or practice sessions?

Recall from chapter 5 that the types of food you choose will vary based on your level of intensity and type of training. What is the intensity of your activity? Is it high (you can't talk), low (you can carry on a conversation), or somewhere between the two? Also, what type of activity are you doing (e.g., strength, endurance)? Your meal skeleton needs to reflect your training type and intensity level. The examples in chapter 5 of fueling for game day may help.

When do you train or practice?

The answer to this question will determine how many times in the day to eat. As you learned in chapter 5, some youth athletes benefit from a preworkout meal and a recovery meal. If your training is over one hour long, you may need to plug in a sport drink or other source of carbohydrate fuel during activity.

When do you eat lunch?

School lunch periods can range from 10:00 a.m. to 1:30 p.m. If you have a 1:30 school lunch, you will need to have a snack at some point in the morning. If you have a 10:00 a.m. lunch period, you may need a snack in the early afternoon.

When do you wake up, and when do you go to bed?

Your first meal of the day should be when you wake up. From that time on, your meals and mini-meals should be evenly spaced throughout the day. When you eat the right food at the right time and in the right amount, you feel energized all day long. You feel better, and your body works better.

Once you have determined your total servings and answered the preceding questions, you are ready to set up your meal skeleton. In my practice, it's not uncommon to meet youth athletes who skip breakfast, eat an enormous lunch, then eat a huge dinner—and that's it. Eating in that way may meet your caloric needs, but it is not necessarily ideal for sport performance. An ideal meal plan involves eating a similar amount of food four or five times per day. Breakfast, lunch, and dinner may be larger, but balanced mini-meals and snacks between those meals help to keep your energy levels maxed out throughout the day. Also, chances are good that your schedule changes from one day to another. Maybe you have practice after school only two nights a week, or your Saturday schedule is far different from your Sunday schedule. Don't worry. A meal skeleton is designed to be flexible.

Figure 8.8 *a* and *b* shows examples of meal skeletons based on two schedules—an early lunch period and a later lunch period. Because practices may fall at different times on different days, you need to learn how to adjust your meals accordingly. Remember that flexibility is the key to success.

In both of these examples, I use the 68-kilogram (150 lb) very active 16-year-old male from earlier figures. Recall from figure 8.6 that we determined his daily servings as follows:

- Carbohydrate: 27
- Protein: 11
- Fat: 23

Figure 8.8a Sample Meal Skeleton: Normal School Lunch Period With After-School Practice

	Time	Place	Starch	Fruit	Nonstarchy vegetable	Milk or yogurt	Other sugar	Protein	Fat	Food example
Meal 1: Breakfast	7:00 a.m.	Home	2	1	0	1	0	4	5	Breakfast sandwich: 2 eggs; 1 oz (30 g) cheese; 2 slices wheat toast; 1 tbsp (15 g) light margarine; 1 cup skim milk ¾ cup blueberries
Meal 2: Lunch	11:00 a.m.	School	3	2	1	1	0	4	4	Grilled chicken sandwich; ½ cup corn (with margarine); 1 cup skim milk; 1 large banana; mixed vegetable salad; 2 tbsp (30 ml) salad dressing

	Time	Place	Starch	Fruit	Nonstarchy vegetable	Milk or yogurt	Other sugar	Protein	Fat	Food example
Meal 3: Prepractice snack	2:30 p.m.	School	2.5	0	0	0	1	1	2	Homemade preworkout energy bar (see high-calorie preworkout bar)
Meal 4: During practice	4:00 p.m.	Practice	0	0	0	0	2	0	0	20 oz (600 ml) sport drink
Meal 5: Recovery snack	5:30 p.m.	Practice	1	1	0	1	1	2	3	8 oz (240 ml) chocolate milk; trail mix: nuts, cereal, dried fruit
Meal 6: Dinner	6:30 p.m.	Home	2	0	1	0	0	3	5	3 oz (90 g) roasted pork; 1 1/2 cups cooked carrots; 1 cup mashed potatoes (with margarine); 2 tsp (10 ml) olive oil
Meal 7: Evening snack	9:30 p.m.	Home	1	0	0	1	1	2	4	5 oz (150 g) flavored Greek yogurt; 1/4 cup granola; 1 oz (30 g) almonds

Figure 8.8b Sample Meal Skeleton: Late School Lunch Period With After-School Practice

	Time	Place	Starch	Fruit	Nonstarchy vegetable	Milk or yogurt	Other sugar	Protein	Fat	Food example
Meal 1: Breakfast	7:00 a.m.	Home	1	2	0	1	1	3	3	2 oz (60 g) ham steak; 1/2 cup oatmeal; 1 tbsp (15 g) brown sugar; 1 cup skim milk; banana; 16 crushed almonds
Meal 2: Midmorning snack	10:00 a.m.	School	1	1	0	0	1	1	4	trail mix: dried fruit, chocolate chips, dried cereal, nuts; 1 oz (30 g) beef jerky
Meal 3: Lunch	1:00 p.m.	School	3	1	0	1	0	3	4	1 cup milk; 1 pulled pork sandwich; 1/2 cup mashed potatoes (with margarine); fruit cup

	Time	Place	Starch	Fruit	Nonstarchy vegetable	Milk or yogurt	Other sugar	Protein	Fat	Food example
Meal 4: During practice	4:00 p.m.	Practice	0	0	0	0	2	0	0	20 oz (600 ml) sport drink
Meal 5: Recovery snack	5:30 p.m.	Practice	2	0	0	0	1	1	2	Homemade recovery bar (see recipe in chapter 11); water
Meal 6: Dinner	6:30 p.m.	Home	3	0	1	1	0	3	5	1 cup pasta; marinara sauce; 1 1/2 cups broccoli; 3 meatballs; 1 breadstick
Meal 7: Evening snack	9:30 p.m.	Home	2	1	0	1	0	2	4	1 oz (30 g) cheese; 10 crackers; 12 grapes; 1 cup skim milk

Now it's time to create your own meal skeleton. In figure 8.9, first, fill in the times that are realistic for you to eat. Remember, not every youth athlete needs a preworkout or recovery snack. Not every youth athlete benefits from a fuel source during activity. Younger athletes need less fuel than older athletes do. Athletes looking to decrease body fat require fewer calories than athletes trying to gain weight. Consider your entire day—your school schedule, training schedule, dinner schedule, bedtime, and everything else—before you start recording. Next, distribute your daily portions across the day.

Figure 8.9   Meal Skeleton Template

	Starch	Fruit	Non-starchy vegetable	Milk or yogurt	Other sugar	Protein	Fat
Meal 1:							
Meal 2:							
Meal 3:							
Meal 4:							
Meal 5:							
Meal 6:							
Meal 7:							

From H.R. Mangieri, 2017, *Fueling young athletes* (Champaign, IL: Human Kinetics).

Step 5: Create a Meal Plan

At this point you know how to categorize food, you have calculated your needs, you have created a meal skeleton that works for you, and you understand the importance of choosing foods from each food group. Now you need to understand one more thing: the foods you choose contain much more than just carbohydrate, protein, and fat. I do not have enough space in this book to explain how to create a meal plan that is 100 percent adequate in every nutrient, every day, nor is that necessary. As noted in chapter 3, nutrient deficiencies do not happen overnight. They can occur when your diet, day after day, is lacking in key nutrients.

If you completed your meal skeleton properly, most meals should look very similar in terms of the amount of food. If you are still eating a small breakfast, medium lunch, and large dinner, you have some work to do on your meal balance. That's OK. Start by eating the foods you love, and strive for balance as you spread them out over the course of the day. Even though you may consider certain foods breakfast foods or snacks, your body does not care. If you eat a handful of pretzels, your body does not know that you ate pretzels. It only knows that you consumed a starchy carbohydrate that will break down to glucose. That's why it is so important to understand serving sizes. If you open a bag of pretzels after school and start mindlessly munching directly from the bag, you can easily eat 2.5 ounces or 75 grams of pretzels, which is equal to 45 grams of carbohydrate or 3 servings of starch, in no time at all. Although the calories in that starchy snack might be adequate, the nutrients are not. Consider that 12 pretzel twists (~2.5 oz, or 75 g) constitute 3 carbohydrate servings. Now compare that to a cup of skim milk, a medium orange, and 18 baby carrots, which combined also constitute 3 carbohydrate portions. Both examples supply a similar number of calories, but the second example provides a lot more nutrients. Not only does it supply a variety of vitamins and minerals, but it also contributes to your daily fiber and protein needs.

Remember, you do not have to change the foods you eat to follow your meal skeleton, but you must adjust your portions (the amount of food you eat). The examples in tables 8.7 to 8.12 are not set up by day but instead by serving sizes per meal. I want to show you how to adjust a meal so that you are eating the amount of food that is right for you. You can use tables 8.7 to 8.12 to build your own meal plan based on your specific portion size needs.

A Note About Rest Days

I am often asked whether caloric intake should be reduced on rest days and increased on training days. The answer depends on a few things. For one, how hungry are you? Just because you are not involved in heavy training one day of the week does not mean that you need less nutrition. Remember, growth and development are not consistent.

Creating a different meal skeleton for every day of the week would be a lot of work and is not necessary. You may need fewer calories on certain days, but the foods you limit should be the lower-nutrient foods, such as sport drinks, beans, or chews, which were there only to support your training. Ideally, you should keep the structure of your day similar and reduce the portions to match your hunger. Maybe you need only one cup of pasta on a rest day but one and a half cups on a day after practice. If you are focused on gaining weight for your sport, you may need to keep your additional snacks and mini-meals in place.

The principle of increasing or reducing portions, not eliminating foods, pertains to feeding an entire family using the same foods. Chances are good that family members have different calorie needs. That does not mean that you make a different meal for each person. It means that people should eat different portions of the same food.

If you are finding it challenging to create your meal skeleton, refer to the examples shown in figure 8.8a and b. The layout and food choices can remain the same, but you may need to adjust the portion sizes at each meal to better meet your individual needs.

Table 8.7 Sample Meal Servings: Breakfast

If your total servings for this meal are . . .	. . . then you can eat this:	Calories (approximate)
2 CHO, 1 PRO, 2 FAT	Balanced breakfast bar (see recipe in chapter 11) (2 CHO + 1 PRO + 2 FAT)	300
2 CHO, 2 PRO, 1 FAT	1/2 cup overnight oats (see recipe in chapter 11) (2 CHO + 1 PRO + 1 FAT) 1 oz (30 g) Canadian bacon or breakfast ham (1 PRO)	275
2 CHO, 2 PRO, 2 FAT	1 slice whole-wheat toast (1 CHO) 3/4 cup blueberries (1 CHO) 1 egg, whole (1 PRO + 1 FAT) 2 egg whites (1 PRO) 1 tbsp (15 g) margarine, light (1 FAT)	350
3 CHO, 3 PRO, 1 FAT	1/2 cup overnight oats (see recipe in chapter 11) (2 CHO + 1 PRO + 1 FAT) 1 cup milk, skim (1 CHO + 1 PRO) 1 oz (30 g) Canadian bacon or breakfast ham (1 PRO)	400
3 CHO, 2 PRO, 2 FAT	2 slices toast, whole wheat (2 CHO) 3/4 cup blueberries (1 CHO) 1 egg, whole (1 PRO + 1 FAT) 2 egg whites (1 PRO) 1 tbsp (15 g) light margarine (1 FAT)	425
3 CHO, 2 PRO, 2 FAT	Balanced breakfast bar (see recipe in chapter 11) (2 CHO +1 PRO + 2 FAT) 1 cup milk, skim (1 CHO + 1 PRO)	425
4 CHO, 4 PRO, 3 FAT	1 cup overnight oats (see recipe in chapter 11) (4 CHO + 2 PRO + 2 FAT) 2 oz (60 g) Canadian bacon or breakfast ham (2 PRO + 1 FAT)	625
4 CHO, 3 PRO, 3 FAT	2 slices toast, whole wheat (2 CHO) 1 banana, large (2 CHO) 2 egg, whole (2 PRO + 2 FAT) 2 egg whites (1 PRO) 1 tbsp (15 g) margarine, light (1 FAT)	575
4 CHO, 3 PRO, 3 FAT	Balanced breakfast bar (see recipe in chapter 11) (2 CHO +1 PRO + 2 FAT) 1 cup milk, skim (1 CHO + 1 PRO) 1 orange (1 CHO) 1 egg, hard-boiled (1 PRO + 1 FAT)	575

If your total servings for this meal are . . .	. . . then you can eat this:	Calories (approximate)
5 CHO, 3 PRO, 5 FAT	1 bagel, large (4 CHO) 3/4 cup blueberries (1 CHO) 2 eggs, whole (2 PRO + 2 FAT) 2 slices sausage, turkey (1 PRO + 2 FAT) 1 tbsp (15 g) margarine, light (1 FAT)	750
5 CHO, 3 PRO, 3 FAT	Balanced breakfast bar (see recipe in chapter 11) (2 CHO +1 PRO + 2 FAT) 1 cup milk, skim (1 CHO + 1 PRO) 1 egg, hard-boiled (1 PRO + 1 FAT) 1 banana, large (2 CHO)	750
5 CHO, 5 PRO, 4 FAT	1 cup overnight oats (see recipe in chapter 11) (4 CHO + 2 PRO + 2 FAT) 3 oz (90 g) Canadian bacon or breakfast ham (3 PRO + 1 FAT) 1 tsp (15 g) peanut butter (add to oats!) (1 FAT) 1/2 cup orange juice (1 CHO)	775

Table 8.8 Sample Meal Servings: Midmorning Mini-Meal or Snack

If your total servings for this meal are . . .	. . . then you can eat this:	Calories (approximate)
1 CHO, 2 PRO, 2 FAT	1/2 turkey sandwich: 1 slice bread, whole wheat (1 CHO) 1 oz (30 g) turkey (1 PRO) 1 oz (30 g) cheese (1 PRO + 2 FAT)	250
1 CHO, 2 PRO, 2 FAT	5.3 oz (150 g) yogurt, Greek (1 CHO + 2 PRO) 10 walnut halves, crushed (2 FAT)	200
2 CHO, 3 PRO, 2 FAT	1/2 turkey sandwich: 1 slice bread, whole wheat (1 CHO) 2 oz (60 g) turkey (2 PRO) 1 oz (30 g) cheese (1 PRO + 2 FAT) 1 orange (1 CHO)	325
2 CHO, 2 PRO, 2 FAT	5.3 oz (150 g) yogurt, Greek (1 CHO + 2 PRO) 2 tbsp (30 g) cranberries, dried (1 CHO) 10 walnut halves, crushed (2 FAT)	330
3 CHO, 2 PRO, 1 FAT	1/2 cup trail mix (see recipe in chapter 11) (2 CHO + 1 PRO + 1 FAT) 1 cup skim or 1% milk (1 CHO + 1 PRO)	330

(continued)

Table 8.8 Sample Meal Servings: Midmorning Mini-Meal or Snack *(continued)*

If your total servings for this meal are . . .	. . . then you can eat this:	Calories (approximate)
3 CHO, 2 PRO, 2 FAT	1/2 cup trail mix (see recipe in chapter 11) (2 CHO + 1 PRO + 1 FAT) 1 cup milk, 2% (1 CHO + 1 PRO + 1 FAT)	375
3 CHO, 3 PRO, 3 FAT	1/2 turkey sandwich: 2 slices bread, whole wheat (2 CHO) 2 oz (60 g) turkey (2 PRO) 1 oz (30 g) cheese (1 PRO + 2 FAT) 1 tsp (5 g) mayo (1 FAT) 12 grapes (1 CHO)	500
3 CHO, 3 PRO, 3 FAT	1 cup yogurt, Greek, plain (1 CHO + 3 PRO) 2 tbsp (30 g) cranberries, dried (1 CHO) 3/4 cup blackberries (1 CHO) 10 walnut halves, crushed (2 FAT) 1 tbsp (15 g) hemp seeds (1 FAT)	500
6 CHO, 3 PRO, 3 FAT	1 cup trail mix (4 CHO + 2 PRO + 2 FAT) 1 cup milk, 2%, flavored (2 CHO + 1 PRO + 1 FAT)	500
4 CHO, 4 PRO, 4 FAT	1 turkey sandwich: 2 slices bread, whole wheat (2 CHO) 3 oz (90 g) turkey (3 PRO) 1 oz (30 g) cheese (1 PRO + 2 FAT) 2 tsp (10 g) mayo (2 FAT) 1 banana, large (2 CHO)	650

Table 8.9 Sample Meal Servings: Lunch

If your total servings for this meal are . . .	. . . then you can eat this:	Calories (approximate)
2 CHO, 3 PRO, 1 FAT	Tacos: 2 taco shells, hard (1 CHO) 2 oz (60 g) beef, ground, 93% lean with spices (2 PRO + 1 FAT) 1 cup skim or 1% milk (1 CHO +1 PRO)	325
2 CHO, 3 PRO, 2 FAT	3 oz (90 g) chicken, grilled (3 PRO) 1 bun, hamburger, small (2 CHO) 2 tsp (10 g) mayo (2 FAT)	375

If your total servings for this meal are . . .	. . . then you can eat this:	Calories (approximate)
2.5 CHO, 3 PRO, 2 FAT	Chicken salad: 2-3 cups greens, mixed (FREE) 1 1/2 cups veggies, raw (0.5 CHO) 3 oz (90 g) chicken, boneless, skinless (3 PRO) 10 French fries, baked (2 CHO + 1 FAT) 2 tbsp salad dressing, light vinaigrette (1 FAT)	415
3 CHO, 3 PRO, 2 FAT	Chicken salad: 2-3 cups mixed greens (FREE) 1 1/2 cups veggies, raw (0.5 CHO) 3 oz (90 g) chicken, boneless, skinless (3 PRO) 13 French fries, baked (2.5 CHO + 1 FAT) 2 tbsp (30 ml) salad dressing, light vinai-grette (1 FAT)	450
3 CHO, 4 PRO, 2 FAT	3 oz chicken, grilled (3 PRO) 1 bun, hamburger, small (2 CHO) 1 oz (30 g) cheese, American (1 PRO + 2 FAT) 1 apple, small (1 CHO)	500
3 CHO, 3 PRO, 3 FAT	Tacos: 2 taco shells, hard (1 CHO) 2 oz (60 g) beef, ground, 93% lean with spices (2 PRO + 1 FAT) 1 oz (30 g) cheese, cheddar (1 PRO + 2 FAT) 1 nectarine (1 CHO) 1 1/2 cups carrots, cooked (1 CHO)	500
3 CHO, 4 PRO, 3 FAT	3 oz (90 g) chicken, grilled (3 PRO) 1 bun, hamburger, small (2 CHO) 1 oz (30 g) cheese, American (1 PRO + 2 FAT) 1 tsp (5 g) mayo (1 FAT) 1 small apple (1 CHO)	575
4 CHO, 5 PRO, 3 FAT	Tacos: 2 taco shells, hard (1 CHO) 2 oz (60 g) beef, ground, 93% lean (3 PRO + 1 FAT) 1 oz (30 g) cheese, cheddar (1 PRO + 2 FAT) 1 cup milk, skim (1 CHO + 1 PRO) 1 nectarine (1 CHO) 1 1/2 cups carrots, cooked (1 CHO)	575

(continued)

Table 8.9   Sample Meal Servings: Lunch *(continued)*

If your total servings for this meal are . . .	. . . then you can eat this:	Calories (approximate)
4 CHO, 4 PRO, 4 FAT	Steak salad: 2-3 cups greens, mixed (FREE) 1 1/2 cups veggies, raw (0.5 CHO) 3 oz (90 g) steak, sirloin (3 PRO + 2 FAT) 13 French fries, baked (2.5 CHO + 1 FAT) 1/2 cup garbanzo beans (1 CHO + 1 PRO) 2 tbsp (30 ml) salad dressing, light vinaigrette (1 FAT)	675
4 CHO, 4 PRO, 3 FAT	3 oz chicken, grilled (3 PRO) 1 bun, hamburger, small (2 CHO) 1 oz (30 g) cheese, American (1 PRO + 2 FAT) 1 small apple (1 CHO) 1 1/2 cups broccoli (1 CHO) 1 tsp (5 ml) olive oil (1 FAT)	750
5 CHO, 5 PRO, 4 FAT	Tacos: 3 taco shells, hard (1.5 CHO) 3 oz (90 g) beef, ground, 93% lean, with spices (3 PRO + 2 FAT) 1 oz (30 g) cheese, cheddar (1 PRO + 2 FAT) 1 banana, medium (1.5 CHO) 1 1/2 cups spinach, cooked (1 CHO) 1 cup milk, skim (1 CHO + 1 PRO)	750
5 CHO, 4 PRO, 4 FAT	Steak salad: 2-3 cups greens, mixed (FREE) 1 1/2 cups veggies, raw (0.5 CHO) 3 oz (90 g) steak, sirloin (3 PRO + 2 FAT) 13 French fries, baked (2.5 CHO + 1 FAT) 1/2 cup garbanzo beans (1 CHO + 1 PRO) 2 tbsp (30 g) cranberries, dried (1 CHO) 2 tbsp (30 ml) salad dressing, vinaigrette (1 FAT)	750

Table 8.10 Sample Meal Servings: After-School Snack

If your total servings for this meal are . . .	. . . then you can eat this:	Calories (approximate)
2 CHO, 2 PRO, 1 FAT	8 oz (240 ml) milk, flavored (2 CHO + 1 PRO) 1 egg, hard-boiled (1 PRO + 1 FAT)	275
3 CHO, 2 PRO, 1 FAT	Roast beef wrap: 1 flour tortilla, small (1 CHO) 2 oz (60 g) roast beef, deli (2 PRO) 2 tbsp (30 g) avocado (1 FAT) Veggies, raw (FREE) 1 banana, large (2 CHO)	375
3 CHO, 2.5 PRO, 1 FAT	12 oz (360 ml) milk, flavored (3 CHO + 1.5 PRO) 1 egg, hard-boiled (1 PRO + 1 FAT)	385
4 CHO, 2 PRO, 1 FAT	1/2 peanut butter and jelly sandwich: 1 slice bread, wheat (1 CHO) 2 tsp (10 g) peanut butter (1 FAT) 1/2 tbsp (8 g) jam (0.5 CHO) 1 banana, medium (1.5 CHO) 1 milk, skim, shelf-stable (1 CHO + 1 PRO) 1 oz (30 g) beef jerky (1 PRO)	450
4 CHO, 2 PRO, 1 FAT	Roast beef wrap: 1 flour tortilla, medium (2 CHO) 2 oz (60 g) roast beef, deli (2 PRO) Veggies, raw (FREE) 1 tbsp (15 g) avocado (1 FAT) 1 banana, large (2 CHO)	450
4 CHO, 3 PRO, 2 FAT	1/2 peanut butter and jelly sandwich: 1 slice bread, wheat (1 CHO) 2 tsp (10 g) peanut butter (1 FAT) 1/2 tbsp (8 g) jelly (0.5 CHO) 1 banana, medium (1.5 CHO) 1 milk, 2%, shelf-stable (1 CHO + 1 PRO + 1 FAT) 2 oz (60 g) beef jerky (2 PRO)	525
4 CHO, 3 PRO, 2 FAT	1 peanut butter and jelly sandwich: 2 slices bread, wheat (2 CHO) 4 tsp (20 g) peanut butter (2 FAT) 1 tbsp (15 g) jelly (1 CHO) 1/2 cup baby carrots, raw (FREE) 1 milk, skim, shelf-stable (1 CHO + 1 PRO) 2 oz (60 g) beef jerky (2 PRO)	525

(continued)

Table 8.10 Sample Meal Servings: After-School Snack *(continued)*

If your total servings for this meal are . . .	. . . then you can eat this:	Calories (approximate)
4 CHO, 3 PRO, 3 FAT	Roast beef wrap: 1 flour tortilla, medium (2 CHO) 2 oz (60 g) roast beef, deli (2 PRO) 1 oz (30 g) cheese (1 PRO + 2 FAT) 2 tbsp (30 g) avocado (1 FAT) 1 banana, large (2 CHO)	525
4 CHO, 3 PRO, 3 FAT	8 oz (240 ml) milk, flavored (2 CHO + 1 PRO) 1/2 pita (1 CHO) Premixed egg salad: 1 egg (1 PRO + 1 FAT) + 2 egg whites (1 PRO) + 2 tsp (10 g) mayonnaise (2 FAT) 1 apple, small (1 CHO)	575
5 CHO, 2.5 PRO, 1 FAT	12 oz (60 g) milk, skim, flavored (3 CHO + 1.5 PRO) 1 egg, hard-boiled (1 PRO + 1 FAT) 16 oz (480 ml) sport drink (2 CHO)	550
5 CHO, 3 PRO, 2 FAT	1 peanut butter and jelly sandwich: 2 slices bread, wheat (2 CHO) 4 tsp (20 g) peanut butter (2 FAT) 1 tbsp (15 g) jelly (1 CHO) 1 banana, small (1 CHO) 1 milk, skim, shelf-stable (1 CHO + 1 PRO) 2 oz (60 g) beef jerky (2 PRO)	625
5 CHO, 4 PRO, 3 FAT	Roast beef wrap: 1 flour tortilla, medium (2 CHO) 2 oz (60 g) roast beef, deli (2 PRO) 1 oz (30 g) cheese (1 PRO + 2 FAT) 2 tbsp (30 g) avocado (1 FAT) 1 banana, large (2 CHO) 1 cup milk, skim (1 CHO + 1 PRO)	650
2 CHO, 2 PRO, 2 FAT	2 meatballs, turkey (see recipe in chapter 11) (2 PRO + 1 FAT) 1/2 cup pasta (1 CHO) 1/4 cup pasta sauce (0.5 CHO) Mixed green salad with raw veggies (0.5 CHO) 2 tbsp (30 ml) salad dressing, light vinaigrette (1 FAT)	325

Table 8.11 Sample Meal Servings: Dinner

If your total servings for this meal are . . .	. . . then you can eat this:	Calories (approximate)
2 CHO, 3 PRO, 2 FAT	3 oz (90 g) chicken breast, boneless, skinless (3 PRO) 3 oz (90 g) potatoes, red skinned (1 CHO) 1 1/2 cups carrots, cooked (1 CHO) 2 tsp (10 ml) oil (to roast potatoes and flavor chicken) (2 FAT)	375
2 CHO, 3 PRO, 2 FAT	3 oz (90 g) Atlantic salmon fillet (3 PRO + 1.5 FAT) 1/3 cup rice, cooked (1 CHO) 1 1/2 cups spinach, cooked (1 CHO) 1/2 tsp (3 ml) olive oil (in spinach) (0.5 FAT)	375
3 CHO, 3 PRO, 2 FAT	3 oz (90 g) chicken breast, boneless, skinless (3 PRO) 3 oz (90 g) potatoes, red skinned (1 CHO) 1 1/2 cups carrots, cooked (1 CHO) 2 tsp (10 ml) oil (to roast the potatoes and flavor chicken) (2 FAT) 1 cup cantaloupe, diced (1 CHO)	450
3 CHO, 3 PRO, 2.5 FAT	3 meatballs, turkey (see recipe in chapter 11) (3 PRO + 1.5 FAT) 2/3 cup pasta (2 CHO) 1/4 cup pasta sauce (0.5 CHO) Mixed green salad with raw veggies (0.5 CHO) 1 1/2 tbsp (23 ml) salad dressing, light vinaigrette (1 FAT)	450
3 CHO, 3 PRO, 2 FAT	3 oz (90 g) Atlantic salmon fillet (3 PRO + 1.5 FAT) 2/3 cup rice, cooked (2 CHO) 1 1/2 cups spinach, cooked (1 CHO) 1/2 tsp (3 ml) olive oil (in spinach) (0.5 FAT)	450
4.5 CHO, 3 PRO, 3.5 FAT	3 meatballs, turkey (see recipe in chapter 11) (3 PRO + 1.5 FAT) 1 cup pasta (3 CHO) 1/2 cup pasta sauce (1 CHO) Mixed green salad with raw veggies (0.5 CHO) 2 tbsp (30 ml) dressing, vinaigrette (2 FAT)	625

(continued)

Table 8.11 Sample Meal Servings: Dinner *(continued)*

If your total servings for this meal are . . .	. . . then you can eat this:	Calories (approximate)
4 CHO, 4 PRO, 3 FAT	4 oz (120 g) chicken breast, boneless, skinless (4 PRO) 6 oz (180 g) potatoes, red skinned (2 CHO) 1 1/2 cups carrots, cooked (1 CHO) 1 cup cantaloupe, diced (1 CHO) 1 tbsp (15 ml) oil (to roast potatoes and flavor chicken) (3 FAT)	625
4 CHO, 4 PRO, 3 FAT	4 oz (120 g) Atlantic salmon fillet (4 PRO + 2 FAT) 1 cup rice, cooked (3 CHO) 1 1/2 cups spinach, cooked (1 CHO) 1 tsp (5 ml) olive oil (in spinach) (1 FAT)	625
5 CHO, 4 PRO, 4 FAT	4 oz (120 g) chicken breast, boneless, skinless (4 PRO) 9 oz (27 g) potatoes, red skinned (3 CHO) 1 1/2 c carrots, cooked (1 CHO) 1 dinner roll, small (1 CHO) 1 tbsp (15 ml) oil (to roast potatoes and flavor chicken) (3 FAT) 1 tsp (5 g) butter (on roll) (1 FAT)	750
5 CHO, 4 PRO, 4 FAT	4 oz (120 g) Atlantic salmon fillet (4 PRO + 2 FAT) 1 cup rice, cooked (3 CHO) 1 1/2 cups spinach, cooked (1 CHO) 1/2 cup corn (1 CHO) 2 tsp (10 ml) olive oil (mixed into veggies) (2 FAT)	750
5 CHO, 4 PRO, 4 FAT	4 meatballs, turkey (see recipe in chapter 11) (4 PRO + 2 FAT) 1 1/2 cups pasta (3 CHO) 1/2 cup pasta sauce (1 CHO) Mixed green salad with raw veggies + 4 croutons (1 CHO) 2 tbsp (30 ml) salad dressing, vinaigrette (2 FAT)	750

Table 8.12 Sample Meal Servings: Evening Mini-Meal or Snack

If your total servings for this meal are . . .	. . . then you can eat this:	Calories (approximate)
1 CHO, 2 PRO, 0 FAT	Basic blueberry smoothie (see recipe in chapter 10)	120
2 CHO, 3 PRO, 0 FAT	Blueberry smoothie (see recipe in chapter 10)	200
2 CHO, 3 PRO, 2 FAT	Chocolate-covered strawberry smoothie (see recipe in chapter 10)	260
3 CHO, 2 PRO, 1 FAT	Green apple, grape, and pineapple smoothie (see recipe in chapter 10)	275
2 CHO, 2 PRO, 2 FAT	2 egg muffins (see recipe in chapter 11) (2 PRO + 2 FAT) 10 oz (300 g) watermelon (1 CHO) 1 bagel, mini (1 CHO)	325
2 CHO, 2 PRO, 2 FAT	Tuna salad on crackers: 6 crackers, round butter type (1 CHO + 1 FAT) 1 oz (30 g) tuna (1 PRO) 1 cup milk, skim (1 CHO + 1 PRO) 1 tbsp (15 g) mayo, light (1 FAT)	325
3 CHO, 2 PRO, 2 FAT	2 egg muffins (see recipe in chapter 11) (2 PRO + 2 FAT) 10 oz (300 g) watermelon (1 CHO) 1/2 bagel, large (2 CHO)	425
3 CHO, 2 PRO, 3 FAT	Tuna salad on crackers: 12 crackers, round butter type (2 CHO + 2 FAT) 2 oz (60 g) tuna (2 PRO) 1 tbsp (15 g) mayo, light (1 FAT) 1 orange (1 CHO)	450
3 CHO, 3 PRO, 3 FAT	Snack platter: 1/2 cup berries (1 CHO) 1/2 cup baby carrots (FREE) 2 oz (60 g) turkey, cubed (2 PRO) 1 oz (30 g) cheese, cubed (1 PRO + 2 FAT) 10 crackers, whole wheat (2 CHO + 1 FAT)	500

(continued)

Table 8.12 Sample Meal Servings: Evening Mini-Meal or Snack *(continued)*

If your total servings for this meal are . . .	. . . then you can eat this:	Calories (approximate)
3 CHO, 3 PRO, 3 FAT	Snack platter: 1 peach (1 CHO) 1 tsp (5 g) nut butter (2 FAT) 1 egg, hard-boiled (1 PRO + 1 FAT) 1/2 cup cottage cheese, 1% fat (2 PRO) 1 cup orange juice (2 CHO)	500
4 CHO, 3 PRO, 4 FAT	2 egg muffins (see recipe in chapter 11) (2 PRO + 2 FAT) 1/4 cup cheese, cheddar, shredded (1 PRO + 2 FAT) 10 oz (300 g) watermelon (1 CHO) 1 bagel, medium (3 CHO)	575
4 CHO, 4 PRO, 3 FAT	Tuna or chicken salad on crackers: 12 crackers, round butter type (2 CHO + 2 FAT) 3 oz (90 g) tuna or chicken (3 PRO) 1 tbsp (15 g) mayo (optional: mixed with 1 tsp, or 5 g, mustard) (1 FAT) 12 grapes (1 CHO) 1 cup milk, skim (1 CHO + 1 PRO)	625
5 CHO, 3 PRO, 4 FAT	2 egg muffins (see recipe in chapter 11) (2 PRO + 2 FAT) 1/4 cup cheese, cheddar, shredded (1 PRO + 2 FAT) 10 oz (300 g) watermelon (1 CHO) 1 bagel, medium (3 CHO) 1/2 cup orange juice (1 CHO)	700
5 CHO, 4 PRO, 4 FAT	Tuna or chicken salad on crackers: 12 crackers, round butter type (2 CHO + 2 FAT) 4 oz (120 g) tuna or chicken (4 PRO) 2 tbsp (30 g) mayo, light (2 FAT) 24 grapes (2 CHO) 1/2 cup apple juice (1 CHO)	725

Though this chapter walks you through the steps to create your own personalized plan, there is a great chance that you feel a bit overwhelmed by the process. Don't panic.

When I work with clients in my office, it is usually not until the third or fourth appointment that they feel capable and confident in creating their own meal plans and swapping foods. And that is with me sitting right by their side. Here, you are trying to learn this material by reading it in a book. You would be the exception if you read this chapter once and felt prepared to put together the perfect meal plan. If you need to, now that you have read through it once, break up the sections and focus on learning them one at a time. Spend one day becoming really familiar with how to categorize foods, and practice that section. Quiz yourself. Once you are feeling confident, move to the next.

Don't expect to read the serving size tables and have them memorized. They are in this book for you to refer back to often. It is not until you have spent time building multiple meal plans that you will begin to remember the specific servings for each food.

Complete the section on calculating your needs once, and then go through the process again. Remember, the numbers are not an exact science. Your calculated needs are an estimate and can be tweaked as necessary based on your hunger, satiety, and goals.

Create a few different meal skeletons and practice by creating a variety of meal plans. The more you practice, the easier it will be and more skilled you will become at putting them together.

If you have worked through the calculations in this chapter and feel satisfied with your meal planning, the next stage is to implement it. If you think developing the plan was a challenge, wait until you see the challenges that you face implementing it. The next chapter shares some strategies you can use to put your nutrition plan into practice while still living your life. I can tell you that it is easier said than done.

Chapter 9

Breaking Down Barriers to Healthy Eating

You now understand nutrition needs and can build a sport nutrition plan. Now comes the hard part: implementing it. Even with the best intentions, life happens. Maybe you don't eat vegetables or dislike protein; maybe you're always on the go and eat most meals out. Whether you're in elementary school, middle school, high school, or college, or are working or raising a family, many things can get in the way of putting a well-designed plan into practice. Succeeding requires some sacrifice from both you and your family.

This chapter shows you how to break down some common barriers to success, even when you're running in 10 directions. Every barrier has a solution; implementing it takes commitment, drive, and flexibility.

Breakfast

You have likely heard that breakfast is the most important meal of the day, and for good reason. Evidence shows that students who eat breakfast have better concentration, attention span, and memory. Studies also show that teenagers who eat breakfast are more likely to take in adequate amounts of iron, the nutrient that helps transport oxygen throughout the body so you stay energized. Skipping this meal also makes it difficult to reach your nutrition needs for the day. Breakfast sets the standard for the day.

Barrier: I would rather sleep than take time for breakfast.

Solution: Grab breakfast to go.

Think outside the box in terms of what breakfast looks like. Prepare and pack foods the night before that you can eat on the way to school or on the bus. Plastic spoons come in handy with some of these breakfasts to go:

- 1/2 cup dry cereal, 2 tbsp (30 g) dried fruit, and 15 nuts in a plastic bag, along with a hard-boiled egg
- A slice of deli ham and a slice of cheese between two halves of a bagel
- 1/2 cup granola and 2 tbsp (30 g) dried fruit in a plastic bag, to dump into a container of Greek yogurt
- Shelf-stable skim milk and a breakfast bar (see chapter 11 for the recipe for a homemade balanced breakfast bar, or purchase a favorite brand)
- 2 string cheeses and a banana

Barrier: I am not hungry in the morning.

Solution: Eat anyway; something is better than nothing.

Your sport nutrition eating plan is part of your training, and hungry or not, that includes breakfast. It does not have to be a sit-down meal of bacon and eggs or a big bowl of oatmeal. If you are not used to eating breakfast, start small. If it is easier, start with liquids! For the first week, commit to having an 8-ounce (240 ml) glass of milk or 12 grapes. It may not be a breakfast of champions (yet!), but it is breakfast. Remember, champions do not determine their future; they determine their habits. Their habits determine their future. Get in the habit of eating breakfast!

Barrier: I can't eat first thing in the morning because I feel nauseated.

Solution: Drink something.

Breakfast does not have to be solid food; liquids can provide nutrition too. If the thought of food first thing in the morning turns your stomach, have a nutritious beverage. Even 4 ounces (120 ml) of milk or juice is better than nothing. Drink that; then grab a breakfast bar to go and eat it as soon as you feel your stomach can tolerate it.

School Lunch

An ideal day for a youth athlete includes a big breakfast before school followed by a well-balanced lunch about four hours later. Unfortunately, that is not always possible. School lunch periods can be as early as 10:00 a.m. and late as 1:30 p.m. Students do not get to choose when they eat lunch in school. This can create challenges for youth athletes trying to eat right at the right time.

Barrier: School lunch is at 10:30 a.m., and practice is directly after school. I'm starving by 2:00 p.m.

Solution: Pack a portable, shelf-stable snack to eat in addition to your school lunch.

Having an earlier lunch period is actually a blessing for youth athletes. That's because eating a mini-meal after school is usually easier than eating one in the middle of the day. If your school lunch is at 10:30 a.m., you should try to have something small between your afternoon classes, ideally around 1:30 or 2:00 p.m. Trail mix, a granola bar, and shelf-stable portable milk are good examples of items you can keep in your locker or backpack and eat quickly before your next class. Some teachers allow students to have foods and beverages in the classroom. If that is the case for you, you can expand your options to something more substantial, such as a peanut butter and jelly sandwich or a yogurt that you have stored in a portable cooler. Either way, you should eat a mini-meal as soon as school ends, around 2:30 p.m. The meal eaten at this time will depend on what you have already eaten and how much time you have before practice.

If you were able to eat a sandwich or yogurt after lunch, then after school you should top off your glycogen stores before practice with something small.

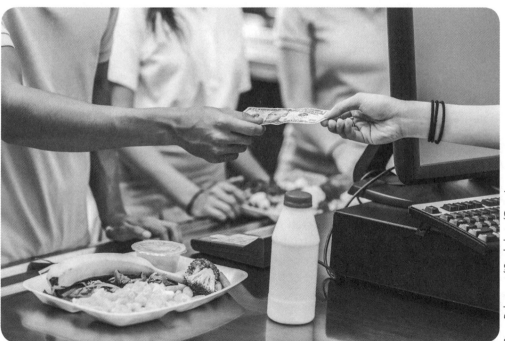

Steve Debenport/iStockphoto/Getty Images

School lunch times can range from 10:00 a.m. to 1:30 p.m. Many young athletes will need a mini-meal at another time during the school day to meet their daily nutrition needs.

If practice starts immediately, at 3:00 or 3:30 p.m., you will need a quick-digesting mini-meal, such as a sport drink, piece of fruit, or preworkout energy bar (see chapter 5 for what to eat when you have only an hour before practice). If practice does not start until 4:00 or 4:30 p.m., you should eat a more balanced mini-meal that includes some protein and healthy fat.

Remember, the key to making your meal plan work for you is flexibility. School lunch times change from year to year. You need to change with them.

Barrier: The school lunch is not enough food for me.

Solution: Purchase two lunches, pack a lunch in addition to your school lunch, or pack a larger lunch.

American schools that participate in the National School Lunch Program offer all students the same calorie range, whether they are athletes or not. That means that a 5-foot 1-inch (155 cm), 110-pound (50 kg) freshman girl is offered the same lunch as the 6-foot 2-inch (188 cm), 170-pound (77 kg) male senior. They can both buy additional items, but that means more money. I have worked with high school athletes who need to eat two or three school lunches to fill up. My point is that the school lunch is not individualized to meet your personal needs. That is your job. To create a meal that fits into your eating plan, you must decide what works for you. That often involves purchasing extra food or bringing food from home.

Barrier: School lunch provides the right amount of protein but exceeds my fat requirements and limits my carbohydrate portions.

Solution: Make adjustments to your selections.

Remember, the standard school lunch meets the needs of the average student. It is not created to meet the extra demands of all hungry high school athletes. To consume all of the portions recommended on your plan, you may need to make adjustments. If you prefer to purchase a lunch, determine how that meal fits into your plan; then pack the additional items needed to reach your recommended portions. From my experience, most of the extra food needed is in the form of complex carbohydrate. Pack an extra piece of fruit, a piece of bread, or pretzels to meet your increased needs. Also, keep in mind that many students fail to eat all of the servings of fruits and vegetables provided in school lunches. As a youth athlete, you need these fruits and vegetables. Make sure you take all of the food you can and that it ends up in your stomach, not the garbage can.

Sport Training and Practice

We talked in previous chapters about the importance of being well fueled before, during, and after training, but doing so takes some extra effort, especially if you have practice before and after school. Even when time is tight, you need to have a plan to fuel your training.

Barrier: My morning practice is at 5:30 a.m., and that is too early to eat.

Solution: Drink a sport drink before practice, and have a portable breakfast after practice.

Although the best plan is to wake up an hour early so you can fuel up before practice, I know that most youth athletes won't do this. The more practical solution is to grab a sport drink as you head out the door and start sipping. Overnight, your glycogen stores have been dwindling, and a sport drink can provide a quick and easily digested source of fuel for your morning workout. But this does not mean that you should skip breakfast. Make sure to fill your mini-cooler with a balanced breakfast that you can eat before you start school. Yogurt cups or tubes; a carton or bottle of milk that you can pour over ready-to-eat cereal; a bagel with peanut butter; and portable protein sources such as cheese cubes, ham slices, hard-boiled eggs, and beef jerky are all good choices.

Barrier: I go directly from school to practice and do not have any time to eat.

Solution: Pack a snack that is nutrient rich and balanced but portable, quick to eat, and quick to digest.

I am a huge advocate of two dinners—one immediately after school and another three or four hours later. Unfortunately, if you go directly to practice after school, you do not have time for a meal. Nevertheless, you need food and nutrition. Suggestions for an after-school meal are a peanut butter and jelly sandwich or peanut butter on crackers; trail mix made with dried cereal, soy nuts, dried fruits, and nuts (see recipe in chapter 11); and a piece of whole fruit. Make sure this mini-meal includes a portable protein such as a few ounces (90 g or so) of turkey, ham, shrimp, yogurt, egg, chicken, or tuna salad (to stuff into a pita). The bigger the break is between school and practice, the more solid your meal can be. The less time you have, the more you may have to rely on liquid nutrition such as milk, yogurt, a sport drink, or a smoothie.

Barrier: I have evening practices and often miss dinner.

Solution: Eat dinner before practice, and be sure to have a recovery meal.

If you created your meal skeleton correctly, most of your meals should provide a balance of carbohydrate, protein, and fat. The only exception is the fuel you take in during exercise. When every meal is balanced, it is easy to move meal-times around to accommodate your schedule. The solution to a late practice may be as easy as eating an early dinner and then a mini-meal after practice.

Barrier: My coach does not allow me to take drink breaks during practice.

Solution: Speak up and express your concern about restricting fuel and fluids.

As a youth athlete, you will be exposed to a variety of coaches, often with very different styles and philosophies. That exposure to different techniques is a big benefit because it helps you learn what works for you. However, when a coach uses abuse techniques to try to get athletes to perform in a certain way, you have every right to speak up. In the scenario described in chapter 3, Mary and I created a hydration schedule that would ensure that she was starting practice well hydrated. I also encouraged Mary's mom to discuss her concerns with the coach and encourage him to allow a few structured drink breaks. Remember, not all coaches are knowledgeable about nutrition and hydration. Unless someone brings a concern to their attention, they may not realize it is a problem. It is OK to speak up.

Homework and Work

No doubt, youth athletes are busy. They are faced with a full day of school, practice and family obligations, and then lots of homework and studying. Some youth athletes also work part-time jobs. Getting all of these things done takes planning and prioritizing.

Barrier: By the time I get to my homework, it is 8:00 at night. I use energy drinks to keep me awake because I get so tired.

Solution: Move healthy hydration and proper fueling to the top of the priority list, and avoid energy drinks.

One of the biggest mistakes of youth athletes is making their meal plan and fluid intake low priorities. As discussed in chapter 6, energy drinks may have the word *energy* in them, but drinking them in the evening to stay awake for homework is counterproductive. Recall the vicious cycle:

energy drink → insomnia → fatigue

Your best bet for meeting your school, training, competition, and homework obligations is getting the right amount of sleep and keeping your body hydrated. Use break times early in the day (e.g., study halls, after-school downtime, car rides) to work on homework. Work ahead on weekend days when you are not as busy. You will have nights that you have to stay up and get the work done. Making your day-to-day nutrition and hydration top priorities is what will help you succeed.

Travel

Traveling with the team is part of the fun, but it can also be a big barrier to following your eating plan. If your sport requires that you travel on the weekends, you may find yourself reliant on whatever food you can find on the way. Like it or not, you are not always in control of where your next meal comes from. I never said being the best is easy. It takes extra thought and extra preparation.

Barrier: I have to eat where the bus stops, and that is often fast food.

Solution: Make the best food choice you can from what is available.

Although it is not ideal, eating out does not have to be a barrier to sticking to your eating plan. Most restaurants, including fast-food establishments, have something healthy on their menus. Order something from the menu that you would eat at home, and be mindful of portions. Table 9.1 gives tips on eating well when traveling with the team.

Barrier: The coach is not thinking about nutrition when selecting a restaurant.

Solution: Take charge and attempt to make a change.

Not all coaches are into nutrition; you might be able to help. Find out who is in charge of selecting the restaurant or bringing foods and drinks for the team, and offer that person suggestions. Before heading to an away game, research the area and suggest healthier restaurants in the area.

Barrier: I have tried to suggest healthier restaurants to my coach, but nothing changes.

Solution: Pack your own food.

If packing your own performance food sounds like a pain, remember this: It is not easy being the best! Grab your mini-cooler and ice packs, and fill the cooler with food from your meal plan. This way you will not be forced to eat when the bus stops but rather when you need and want to eat. (See figure 5.1 in chapter 5, the athlete's portable pantry, for more ideas on what to pack for weekend travel.) Additionally, this allows you to pack other snacks to eat throughout the day, including the right recovery meal.

Barrier: I am tired of always eating granola bars, trail mix, fruit, and yogurt. I wish I could eat a hot meal while I am traveling.

Solution: Pack a hot meal!

You absolutely can pack hot meals to take with you when traveling. Most restaurants will heat up your meal for you. The exception is fast-food restaurants and airport restaurants; you should assume that they will not be willing to heat your meal. Most convenience stores have a microwave you can use to heat up a hot meal. This may seem like a big inconvenience, but eventually it turns into just what you do.

Sleep

Your body works hard for you all day long. By evening, it deserves a rest. Sleep is your body's opportunity to recover. As you fall into a deep sleep, your body becomes more relaxed, slows down, and heals. When you give your body the

Table 9.1 Tips for Eating Well When Traveling

Scenario	What to do
Continental breakfast is the only option at the hotel.	Limit simple sugar and high-fat strudels, doughnuts, and Danishes. Grab a bagel, whole-wheat toast or English muffin, and some peanut butter and jelly. Have dry cereal with milk, a piece of fruit, or oatmeal. Some continental breakfast bars have hot foods. Have a hard-boiled egg or yogurt to meet your protein needs. Think ahead! Grab a few items to take with you as a mini-meal for later.
Breakfast from a service station or mini-mart is the only option.	Look for single-serve cereal, and eat it with milk and a piece of fruit. Look in the refrigerator section for hard-boiled eggs, cheese, or yogurt cups. You might be able to find a hot breakfast sandwich, but beware. They may be much higher in fat than you want. A breakfast bar is also an option, but make sure to read the label.
Breakfast at a fast-food establishment is the only option.	A breakfast burrito is a good selection at a fast-food place. Don't be afraid to customize your order. If English muffins or bagels are offered in a sandwich form (e.g., egg, bacon, and cheese sandwich), you can order a plain bagel or English muffin and add some peanut butter and jelly. Nowadays, most fast-food restaurants offer some variety of fruit. Have that with milk, and you walk away with a fat-controlled breakfast.
You're in a car and do not want to stop.	Invest in a travel-size cooler and a few ice packs. Fill the cooler with meals and snacks for the day, and carry it with you in the car or on the airplane. Bring plenty of water or other beverage (but not sugar filled) to stay hydrated. Nuts such as almonds, cashews, and walnuts mixed with dried fruit are easy to take on a trip in either individual bags or larger containers.
You're staying in a hotel and need snacks between breakfast, lunch, and dinner.	Find a local grocery store and buy healthy snack items such as fruit and nuts or healthy choices from a salad bar or deli section. If your hotel has a refrigerator or microwave, you can buy healthy frozen dinners or soups. If your only choice for a snack is the hotel vending machine, skip the candy and chips and look for nuts or crackers.
Your only options for lunch and dinner are fast food.	Find sandwich shops that let you select your sandwich ingredients. Choose whole-grain breads, lean meats, and lots of vegetables. Many fast-food restaurants offer salads, but you need to be careful. Some are very high in fat, especially taco salads and those topped with fried chicken strips. Order sandwiches made with grilled chicken rather than fried chicken. If you are looking for healthy carbohydrate choices, try a fast-food restaurant that offers baked potatoes or baked chips as sides rather than high-fat French fries. Do not use eating out as an excuse to overeat. Choose foods that are prepared the way you would prepare them at home. Select beverages that you would drink at home.

rest it needs and deserves, it will work well for you. That's why getting a good night's sleep should be a priority. Depriving your body of sleep can limit your ability to learn, listen, and focus, which can negatively affect your performance in the classroom and in your sport. It can leave you in a bad mood and lead to aggressive behavior. It can also lead to poor food choices. A study suggested that sleep deprivation appeared to be associated with injuries in the adolescent athletic population. (Milewski, 2014) Specifically, athletes who slept on average less than eight hours per night were 1.7 times more likely to suffer an injury than did athletes who slept for eight or more hours.

For many youth athletes, getting enough sleep is challenging. As children progress into middle and high school, the school day starts earlier and the work load increases. Tack on sport training and a developing social life, and watch sleep slide down the priority list. Even without sports, the myriad of changes that occur during the adolescent years can easily affect the ability to sleep.

To improve your chances of getting a good night's sleep, the U.S. National Sleep Foundation suggests the following:

- Stick to a sleep schedule, even on the weekends.
- Do not leave homework for the last minute. Try to schedule homework and study opportunities into the day.
- If needed, practice a relaxing bedtime ritual.
- Exercise daily. (Youth athletes have this covered!)
- Beware of things that may disrupt sleep, such as consuming energy drinks.
- Set up a sound sleep environment: Set a comfortable temperature and make sure the sound and light are appropriate for you.
- Use a comfortable pillow and mattress.
- Turn off all electronics. (You may want to consider leaving them in a different room.)

Family Differences

When two of my kids were in third and fifth grades, they both had early school lunch periods and came home from school extremely hungry. They did not need an after-school snack; they needed a meal. My solution was to serve dinner at 4 p.m. and then a mini-meal around 7:00 p.m. Between dinner and the evening mini-meal was swimming practice, gymnastics, religious education, and my third son's therapy (he has severe autism, so his evenings are filled with therapy rather than sports). Every day was go-go-go! I was lucky enough to have a flexible job so that I could be home when my kids got off the bus. However, not all parents are. Whether your kids go to after-school care, stay after school for practice, or go home to a babysitter, they need a balanced meal. It might be a mini-meal, but it is still a meal. If kids are not taught to eat meals when they are hungry, they will fill up on quick snacks.

Remember the discussion in chapter 1 about what makes a star athlete: Champions do not decide their future. Champions decide their habits. Their habits decide their future.

This year, things changed. My fourth-grade daughter eats lunch early, but my sixth-grade son eats lunch later. That means that she comes home hungry, but he doesn't. My solution is to feed my daughter dinner at 3:45 p.m. and then heat my son's dinner a little later, around 4:30 p.m. My third son has difficulty gaining weight, so he eats on a very structured schedule. His mealtimes fall at 3:30 and 7:00 p.m.

So, what do you do when kids are on different schedules? You get flexible. Sometimes even in the same family, meal skeletons (patterns) have to be set up differently. That is the reality of a sporting family! Having multiple kids running in multiple directions is often a reality, but it does not mean that the family's health has to be sacrificed.

Barrier: The kids are very hungry as soon as they get home, but I can't make dinner that quickly.

Solution: Bulk-cook ahead of time.

Open my refrigerator on a Monday, and you would think I was ready to feed an army. That's because I take three to five hours on Sunday evenings to pre-pare and cook seven or eight full meals for the week. I use all of my kitchen resources to make it work: slow cooker, oven, stovetop, microwave—even my outside grill is getting action. I chop and dice vegetables for the week, and I clean and cut up fruit so it is ready to go. Everything goes into glass containers in the refrigerator. This works for us because between homework and extracurricular activities, I do not have time to cook a healthy meal every night.

Take a minute to think about the foods you visualize when you hear the word *snack*? For many kids, the word refers to a quick, often salty, crunchy food (e.g., popcorn or chips) to eat to stave off hunger. Snack foods can fill kids up quickly, but many do not provide proper nourishment.

Having meals ready in the refrigerator prevents kids from grabbing low-nutrient snacks to satisfy their after-school hunger. Get them in the habit of eating a healthy meal; then they can have a balanced mini-meal later in the day.

Barrier: I have no time to cook during the week, and on the weekends we are always traveling for my daughter's traveling league.

Solution: Plan ahead and get creative.

When it comes to eating well, options other than spending lots of time in the kitchen are available. Here are a few examples:

- *Use a slow cooker.* A slow cooker is the answer to a busy family's prayers! Before you leave for work in the morning, toss all of the ingredients in the cooker, turn it on, and go to work. When you get home, the meal is ready. You will need to do some prep work the evening before. I recommend having everything ready to go so that the morning is as easy as possible. Clean and trim chicken, have potatoes cleaned and ready to cut, chop vegetables, and so on. If you are adding spices, have them measured and ready to add to the dish.

- *Stop for a healthy fast-food meal.* Eating out is a reality for many busy sport families, and that is OK. Today, it is possible to find a healthy option at most restaurants, even fast-food establishments. Table 9.1 earlier in this chapter offers tips for eating well when traveling. Those same foods can be used when the travel is only from school to practice.

- *Load up your cooler and take your food with you.* If you cooked in advance as I suggested, this is a time to cash in on your preparations. Grab a few of those homemade meals from the freezer, put them in a cooler, add a few ice packs, and off you go.

- *Have a frozen meal.* I don't often encourage frozen meals (unless they are homemade), but busy times call for easy solutions. If you have a favorite frozen meal or entrée that you know your youth athlete will eat, keep a few in the freezer as a backup. On a day when all else fails, that frozen meal is better than nothing at all.

Barrier: I make a healthy dinner, but my kids won't eat it.

Solution: Serve two dinners; or serve the meal before they fill up on snacks.

A major complaint from parents is that their kids will not eat what they make for dinner. If kids are filling up on low-nutrient snacks after school (e.g., chips, cookies, crackers), when dinnertime rolls around, they may not be hungry for your well-balanced meal. Forget snacks; youth athletes need meals. Serve the meal first.

Barrier: All of my kids are picky and like different foods.

Solution: Offer choices.

Just like adults, kids and teens have likes and dislikes. They also strive for control (some more than others). One way to help them have control is to offer food choices—not 10 choices, but 2. Cooking meals in advance makes this very easy because the food is already in the refrigerator. Think of a meal that is well accepted by most members of the family, and have it available. For example, I always have turkey burgers in my refrigerator. If my son does not like the meal I prepared for dinner, I allow him to heat up a turkey burger and have it with a side of fruit and vegetables.

Barrier: My kids always complain about what I make for dinner.

Solution: Create a meal rotation.

It would be nice if kids just ate what was made for dinner every night, but that is not the reality. As a parent, you have the benefit of not buying or cooking food that you do not like; kids are not so lucky. It is important for kids to try new foods and eat a variety, but it is not necessarily fair that you get to make all the decisions. To increase the chances that your kids will eat what you cook, involve them in the process. Children like to be included in decisions, and it helps them learn about food, nutrition, and meal planning. Have them help you create a meal rotation for the week that includes their favorites. Have each member of the family choose a day of the week and write down what he or she wants to eat that day. When one child complains that she doesn't want to eat that, you can remind her that it is not her night to choose, and that another night everyone will have to eat her selection. With everyone's help, the weekly menu is made.

If everyone agrees, the meals can be simple and repeat weekly. Have the family decide on five meals that everyone loves, such as spaghetti and meatballs, tacos, stir-fry, chili, and sandwiches. During the busy season, rotate through these meals if necessary. The goal is to eat a healthy, balanced meal without causing stress to the chef.

Family Meal

As parents, we make a lot of sacrifices to help our kids succeed—so much so that their basic needs can get lost. One day, you will look back on all of this craziness and wonder how you did it. You will probably miss it, too. Although it seems impossible at times, time together as a family is important for the emotional well-being of children. A very important behavior occurs in the home environment that deserves to be moved to the top of the priority list. That behavior is shared mealtimes.

Although your teen might roll his eyes at you for insisting on eating as a family, one day this shared experience will be what he remembers the most. Sitting down as a family and discussing topics outside of sports help your athlete realize that she is more to you than an athlete; she is a child whom you love and support. Evidence supports this for several reasons. More frequent family meals are associated with a greater consumption of healthy foods in children, adolescents, and adults and may decrease the risk of overweight and obesity in children and adolescents. This shared experience may also protect against eating disorders and other negative behaviors. Shared family meals improve the perception of the family relationship, leaving kids and teenagers feeling safe and cared for.

Barrier: All three of my kids play different sports and have different practice times. A family meal will not work.

Solution: Think outside the normal definition of a meal.

A meal does not have to be hot; maybe it is at 7:30 in the evening when you all sit around to a structured mini-meal (i.e., a balanced snack). Maybe dad is eating a bigger dinner, but mom is simply sipping hot tea. Not all families are able to sit down to a dinner together. For busy sport families, a family meal might have to be at 6:30 in the morning or it might have to be at 8:30 at night. It might be at the ball field on a blanket or at a restaurant after a sporting event. The important thing is that the family be together.

On some days, family meals may not work at all. That's OK, too. If Sunday evening or Monday morning is the only time the family is together, make that the family meal. The important thing is that children and teenagers perceive this behavior as important and know that keeping the family together at times is a priority.

Barrier: My family is never home at the same time.

Solution: Schedule a family meal or date night.

Research supports the value of frequent family meals, but work and practice schedules do not always make that easy. If you cannot make this happen daily, do not stress about it. If possible, set aside 15 to 20 minutes each day to gather the family to talk about the day. The important thing is that kids perceive family time as important to you. In the meantime, schedule a family date night. Maybe you all block off a Sunday afternoon to go bowling or schedule a lunch date. Just make sure that this family time does not get moved to the bottom of the priority list. If something gets scheduled within that time, make that, not the family, wait. You may be shocked at how much respect you receive when you say, "I can't make it; I have a date with my family."

Barrier: I do not know what to cook because my kids have different goals. My daughter needs to lose weight, but my son is trying to gain weight.

Solution: Cook the same foods; just make adjustments.

Having family members with different nutrition needs and goals does not mean that you can't all enjoy a meal together. It just means that at your family meal, not everyone will eat the same amount of food. Each person just needs to stick to his or her individual portion sizes. For example, a younger athlete might require only half a cup of mashed potatoes, whereas an older athlete trying to gain weight might need two cups. Even with increased portion sizes, the calories may need to be higher. You can do this by adding extras. For example, mix a teaspoon (5 ml) of olive oil into the mashed potatoes to bulk up the calories. Refer to chapter 4 for other tips for gaining weight.

Another idea is to cook the same foods, but prepare them different ways. This is more work for the chef, but it can make the meal work for everyone. For example, if you are preparing a chicken casserole dish, top only half of the casserole with cheese. Those trying to limit dietary fat and calories can eat from the side without cheese, and those who need the extra calories can get them from the extra cheese. The other option is to prepare the casserole in two 8- by 8-inch (20 by 20 cm) pans instead of one 9- by 13-inch (23 by 33 cm) pan. Having two separate dishes means that you can use different sauces, protein sources, and so on.

Money

Eating more food, especially high-quality food, can result in a higher grocery bill, and that is a huge barrier for many families. Luckily, many of the extra foods that growing athletes need are not too expensive. Complex carbohydrate sources such as grains, pasta, oatmeal, and other cereals can be purchased in bulk and are relatively inexpensive compared to other foods. High-quality protein is the most expensive nutrient, but putting the strategies discussed in this book into practice will result in eating smaller portions of protein at each meal. This will both improve nutritional efficiency and save money. This section addresses some financial barriers and some tips on overcoming them.

Barrier: I have three athletic teenagers who are eating me out of the house. My grocery bill is outrageous.

Solution: Create a grocery list based on your weekly meal rotation, and stick to it!

Food is expensive. Trying to feed a large family on a budget can get overwhelming if you do not plan ahead and stick to your plan. Make sure to create a weekly meal plan and take the time to record the ingredients needed for the week. Buying lots of extras (snack foods that are eaten quickly and mindlessly) can add hundreds of dollars to your weekly bill, and they tend to be the foods that disappear the fastest. That can also result in the meals you prepare not being eaten, leaving you feeling as though you wasted your time and money making the meal. Make sure to fill your cart with nourishing foods that will be eaten to satisfy hunger, not necessarily because they taste so yummy.

Barrier: Eating healthy food is expensive.

Solution: When possible, choose store brands over popular brands.

The label of the store brand option may not look fancy, but the nutrition value is most likely the same. Many store-brand foods are purchased from companies that make the name-brand foods you love; they are offered at reduced prices because they are not as pretty. Take French fries, for example. A bag of your favorite brand probably contains frozen potato strips that all look very similar in width and length. Consumers tend to prefer this uniformity. Open the store-brand version, and you will likely see different shapes and lengths. These French fry "rejects" are not less nutritious than the pretty French fries in the brand-name bag; they just look different.

Barrier: My kids are always hungry; all of the food I buy is gone by Thursday, and I cannot afford to buy double the amount.

Solution: Buy in bulk.

Buying food in single-serve containers is certainly convenient, but it is also expensive. Instead, buy food in bulk when possible. Buying in bulk does means more money up front, but you can save a lot over the course of a month.

Barrier: If I buy in bulk, my kids just eat more.

Solution: Transfer bulk food into single-serve containers.

Hungry adolescents don't spend much time considering the hunger status of others in the family; they tend to worry only about themselves. How many times have you found an empty cardboard box in your cabinet because someone snatched the last item but didn't consider throwing the box away? Buying in bulk saves money and time if it does not result in the kids' unnecessarily doubling their portion sizes. To keep the convenience of the single-serves while still saving money, transfer bulk foods into single-serve containers as soon as you get home from shopping. Busy teens see portioning out their own food as a hassle (and they are right!). Taking the bulk shopping one step further increases the chances that they will eat the right amount of food.

Barrier: Fresh fruits and vegetables are expensive.

Solution: Buy frozen.

Frozen vegetables are just as nutritious as fresh vegetables and will likely last longer. Frozen vegetables are often sold in convenient steamer bags that allow you to simply pull from the freezer and microwave. As with other single-serve containers, you have to pay for that convenience. I recommend buying bags of frozen vegetables in bulk and preparing only the amount you want to serve for that meal. All you have to do is pour the frozen vegetables into a microwave-safe dish, add a few tablespoons of water and a drizzle of olive oil, and steam for 10 to 15 minutes (depending on the amount you are preparing.) The rest of the bag will stay fresh in the freezer, eliminating food waste.

Fruit can be purchased frozen, too, especially if it is being used in smoothies or pureed for fruit sauces. Fruits such as bananas and apples are less expensive when purchased fresh in bulk.

Barrier: I have two high school athletes who drink one or two bottles of sport drink each day with their training. I can't afford it.

Solution: Make a homemade sport drink.

A 20 oz, or 600 ml, bottle of commercial available sport drink costs over $1.00 (U.S.) per bottle. If you have multiple athletes drinking one or more a day, the cost can add up very quickly. Instead of buying a name brand, you can make the same 20-ounce (600 ml) drink at home for under $0.25. Start saving your favorite sport bottles, make a batch of homemade sport drinks, and pour them into the bottles so that they are ready to grab and go.

Barrier: Even when I am mindful of portion sizes, high-quality protein is expensive. The leaner portions tend to be even more expensive than the higher-fat versions.

Solution: Choose less expensive types of protein.

Protein is expensive compared to the other macronutrients, but you can save money by choosing the right options. Have a variety of choices in your weekly meal plan, including plant-based protein found in beans and legumes. Other less expensive protein choices are milk, canned tuna, eggs, whey protein, cottage cheese, and yogurt. Get creative with these products by using them in meals. You can easily reach the recommendation of 20 to 30 grams of protein without eating a meat-based meal. Try the following to boost protein with meat:

- Top bean-based chili with cheese and serve it with a glass of milk.
- Make pancakes with cottage cheese (see recipe in chapter 11).
- Top whole-wheat pasta with half a cup of cottage cheese instead of meat sauce.
- Make egg muffins. (See recipe in chapter 11; they are only $0.25 per muffin.)
- Make a cottage cheese and fruit plate.
- Mash half a cup of white beans on a whole-wheat wrap and add vegetables and avocado.
- Make a meal-replacement shake with whey protein.

Implementing a sport nutrition plan requires sacrifice from both the family and the athlete. I shared some strategies for overcoming barriers, and you will surely run into some not mentioned here. Be flexible and creative, and you will surely succeed at breaking down the barriers you face.

Part IV

Recipes

Chapter 10

Liquid-Fuel Recipes

Sometimes, liquid fuel is better tolerated than solid fuel. Some athletes simply prefer liquids, and others use it to add extra calories without more volume. This chapter provides ideas and recipes for a variety of fluid-based, easily digested fueling options such as smoothies and sport drinks.

Smoothies

Smoothies are a quick way to get high-quality nutrients between meals. The trick is to make them taste good while keeping them nutritionally balanced. Your meals and mini-meals, whether served on a plate or in a glass, should contain a combination of healthy carbohydrate, high-quality protein, and some healthy fat. Table 10.1 can be used as a guide for building a balanced smoothie.

Choose only one serving from each category. A smoothie that has a banana, 3/4 cup berries, and a mango may taste good, but would you ever eat that much fruit at one time if it was served on a plate? It is important to have the same balance in the blender as you would have on your plate. Here are some other tips to help you make great smoothies.

- For a postworkout smoothie, aim for a ratio of 3:1 to 4:1 carbohydrate to protein; this is optimal for recovery. This chapter includes a few balanced smoothie recipes. You can also use the recipes as a guide and swap out the fruit to change the flavor.
- If you use frozen fruit, purchase varieties with no added sugar.
- Be aware of the fat content of your liquid base and protein; try to choose low-fat or fat-free varieties.
- You can adjust the consistency of the smoothie by adding more liquid or using fruits and vegetables that are less dense.
- Be creative! This formula guarantees a nutritionally balanced smoothie, so throw your taste buds some (delicious) curveballs!

Table 10.1　How to Build a Balanced Smoothie

Choose a base (1/2 to 1 cup)	Choose a fruit (1 to 2 cups)	Choose a vegetable (1 to 2 cups)	Choose a protein (amount varies)	Choose a fat (amount varies)	Additions (amount varies)
*100% fruit juice *Almond drink (milk) *Brewed tea *Coconut water *Milk *Rice beverage *Soy milk *Water	Apple Banana Blackberries Blueberries Cherries Grapes Kiwi Mango Melon Orange Papaya Peach Pear Pineapple Raspberries Strawberries	Beet greens Butternut squash Carrots Celery Collard greens Cucumbers Kale Pumpkin Spinach Sweet potato	Cottage cheese Greek yogurt Protein powder Silken tofu	Avocado (1/4) Chia seeds (1-2 tbsp, or 15-30 g) Chopped nuts (1/8 cup) Ground flaxseed (1-2 tbsp, or 15-30 g) Hemp seeds (1-2 tbsp, or 15-30 g) Nut butter (1 tbsp, or 15 g)	Cocoa powder Fish oil Flavor extracts Herbs and spices Honey Ice Wheat germ

Following are six smoothie recipes with ingredient lists, instructions, nutrition facts, and portion sizes so that you know exactly how to fit them into your meal plan.

Chocolate-Covered Strawberry Smoothie

2 CHO + 3 PRO + 2 FAT

1 cup milk, nonfat, with vitamins A and D

9 strawberries, frozen, unsweetened

1 tbsp (15 g) peanut butter, creamy

1/2 scoop (~15 g) whey protein powder, chocolate

Chocolate chips (a few for garnish)

Add all ingredients to a blender and blend until smooth. Top with chocolate chips.

Nutrition Facts

1 serving per container
Serving size 1 smoothie (372g)

Amount per serving
Calories 260

% Daily Value*

Total Fat 8g	**12%**
Saturated Fat 1.5g	**8%**
Trans Fat 0g	
Cholesterol 5mg	**2%**
Sodium 240mg	**10%**
Total Carbohydrate 26g	**9%**
Dietary Fiber 3g	**12%**
Total Sugars 18g	
Includes 0g Added Sugars	
Protein 23g	
Vitamin D 2.5mcg	17%
Calcium 332mg	35%
Iron 2.85mg	15%
Potassium 141mg	3%

* The % Daily Value (DV) tells you how much a nutrient in a serving of food contributes to a daily diet. 2,000 calories a day is used for general nutrition advice.

Blueberry Smoothie

2 CHO + 3 PRO + 0 FAT

3/4 cup blueberries, frozen

6 oz (180 g) yogurt, Greek, nonfat, vanilla

2 oz (60 ml) milk, nonfat, with vitamins A and D

Add all ingredients to a blender and blend until smooth.

Nutrition Facts

1 serving per container
Serving size 1 smoothie (332g)

Amount per serving
Calories 190

% Daily Value*

Total Fat 1g	**2%**
Saturated Fat 0g	**0%**
Trans Fat 0g	
Cholesterol 0mg	**0%**
Sodium 100mg	**4%**
Total Carbohydrate 29g	**10%**
Dietary Fiber 3g	**12%**
Total Sugars 25g	
Includes 0g Added Sugars	
Protein 19g	
Vitamin D 0.7mcg	5%
Calcium 270mg	25%
Iron 0mg	0%
Potassium 395mg	8%

* The % Daily Value (DV) tells you how much a nutrient in a serving of food contributes to a daily diet. 2,000 calories a day is used for general nutrition advice.

Basic Blueberry Smoothie

1 CHO + 2 PRO + 0 FAT

1/2 cup blueberries, frozen

4 oz (120 g) yogurt, Greek, nonfat, plain

2 oz (60 ml) milk, nonfat, with vitamins A and D

Add all ingredients to a blender and blend until smooth.

Nutrition Facts

1 serving per container

Serving size 1 smoothie (240g)

Amount per serving

Calories 120

	% Daily Value*
Total Fat 0.5g	1%
Saturated Fat 0g	0%
Trans Fat 0g	
Cholesterol 0mg	0%
Sodium 75mg	3%
Total Carbohydrate 16g	5%
Dietary Fiber 2g	8%
Total Sugars 13g	
Includes 0g Added Sugars	
Protein 14g	
Vitamin D 0.7mcg	5%
Calcium 203mg	20%
Iron 0mg	0%
Potassium 293mg	6%

* The % Daily Value (DV) tells you how much a nutrient in a serving of food contributes to a daily diet. 2,000 calories a day is used for general nutrition advice.

Green Smoothie

3 CHO + 2 PRO + 1 FAT

1/2 cup grapes, fresh green

1/3 cup yogurt, Greek, nonfat, plain

1 1/2 cups baby spinach, fresh

1/2 apple, large

1/3 cup pineapple chunks, fresh

1 tbsp (15 g) hemp seeds

Add all ingredients to a blender with 1 cup of ice. Blend until smooth. For a thinner juice, add water.

Nutrition Facts

1 serving per container

Serving size 1 smoothie (374g)

Amount per serving

Calories 260

	% Daily Value*
Total Fat 4g	6%
Saturated Fat 0g	0%
Trans Fat 0g	
Cholesterol 0mg	0%
Sodium 90mg	4%
Total Carbohydrate 46g	15%
Dietary Fiber 6g	24%
Total Sugars 33g	
Includes 0g Added Sugars	
Protein 12g	
Vitamin D 0mcg	0%
Calcium 107mg	10%
Iron 3mg	15%
Potassium 334mg	7%

* The % Daily Value (DV) tells you how much a nutrient in a serving of food contributes to a daily diet. 2,000 calories a day is used for general nutrition advice.

Beetroot Smoothie

2 CHO + 0 PRO + 0 FAT

1 tbsp (15 g) beet crystals, red

4 oz (120 ml) pineapple juice

1/2 cup pineapple chunks, fresh

Add all ingredients to blender with ice to desired consistency. Blend until smooth.

Nutrition Facts

1 serving per container
Serving size 1 smoothie (206g)

Amount per serving
Calories 140

% Daily Value*

Total Fat 0g	**0%**
Saturated Fat 0g	**0%**
Trans Fat 0g	
Cholesterol 0mg	**0%**
Sodium 5mg	**0%**
Total Carbohydrate 33g	**11%**
Dietary Fiber 1g	**4%**
Total Sugars 25g	
Includes 11g Added Sugars	
Protein 1g	
Vitamin D 0mcg	0%
Calcium 11mg	2%
Iron 2.25mg	10%
Potassium 232mg	5%

* The % Daily Value (DV) tells you how much a nutrient in a serving of food contributes to a daily diet. 2,000 calories a day is used for general nutrition advice.

Chocolate Peanut Butter Smoothie

2 CHO + 3 PRO + 2 FAT

1 tbsp (15 g) peanut butter, creamy

1/2 banana, medium

1 tbsp (15 g) cocoa powder, unsweet-ened, natural

1/2 scoop (~15 g) whey protein powder, chocolate

1/2 cup milk, nonfat, with vitamins A and D

1 cup baby spinach, fresh

Add all ingredients to a blender with 1/2 cup of ice. Blend until smooth.

Nutrition Facts

1 serving per container
Serving size 1 smoothie (242g)

Amount per serving
Calories 270

% Daily Value*

Total Fat 10g	**15%**
Saturated Fat 2g	**10%**
Trans Fat 0g	
Cholesterol 15mg	**5%**
Sodium 190mg	**8%**
Total Carbohydrate 30g	**10%**
Dietary Fiber 6g	**24%**
Total Sugars 15g	
Includes 0g Added Sugars	
Protein 22g	
Vitamin D 1.47mcg	10%
Calcium 255mg	25%
Iron 1.7mg	10%
Potassium 515mg	11%

* The % Daily Value (DV) tells you how much a nutrient in a serving of food contributes to a daily diet. 2,000 calories a day is used for general nutrition advice.

Sport Drinks

Sport drinks are the simplest form of liquid fuel that youth athletes can make. They can be included on days when they have back-to-back competitions or used as a fuel source before, during, or after exhaustive exercise. Recall that sport drinks are designed to replace fluid and sodium losses as well as provide some simple fuel for working muscles. A sport drink that is designed properly (i.e., has a proper concentration of fluid, carbohydrate, and sodium) absorbs rapidly, causes little or no gastrointestinal distress, and enhances exercise performance.

The nutrition facts of the following recipes are the same as or close to what you would find in the popular sport drink brands on the market. What they do not have is added color or artificial flavors. The recipes showcase a variety of ways to reach the optimal concentrations, but these drinks do not taste the same as many of the popular brands on the market. You can create your own variety of sport drink by adding calorie-free flavorings. A variety of products for flavoring water are on the market today. Just be mindful of what you add: Increasing the sugar content of a sport beverage above the 5 to 8 percent carbohydrate solution can cause gastrointestinal distress.

Over the years, I have asked athletes what they like and dislike about commercial sport drinks. Some find them too sweet; some dislike the artificial ingredients; others find them too expensive. Athletes who wear face masks worry about spilling and staining their uniforms; they want clear beverages.

Some athletes believe that coconut water is a good sport beverage. Unfortunately, coconut water does not compare nutritionally to other sport beverages because it does not have the concentration of carbohydrate and sodium required to properly replace losses. If you like the taste of coconut water, you can add flavored coconut water to one of the following recipes to make a sport drink that has coconut flavor.

For less than a dollar, coaches can use the 3-quart recipe to make a homemade sport drink for the team.

2 CHO + 0 PRO + 0 FAT

19 oz (570 ml) water

7 tsp (35 g) sugar, white, granulated

1/8 tsp (0.6 g) table salt

1 tbsp (15 ml) lime juice

Heat 1 cup of water in a microwave. Add the hot water to a pitcher, and dissolve the sugar and salt. Add the lime juice and remaining water. Pour into a 20-ounce (600 ml) bottle and chill.

Nutrition Facts

1 serving per container

Serving size   20 ounce bottle (584g)

Amount per serving

Calories 120

% Daily Value*

Total Fat 0g	**0%**
Saturated Fat 0g	**0%**
Trans Fat 0g	
Cholesterol 0mg	**0%**
Sodium 310mg	**13%**
Total Carbohydrate 29g	**10%**
Dietary Fiber 0g	**0%**
Total Sugars 29g	
Includes 29g Added Sugars	
Protein 0g	
Vitamin D 0mcg	0%
Calcium 17mg	2%
Iron 0mg	0%
Potassium 15mg	0%

* The % Daily Value (DV) tells you how much a nutrient in a serving of food contributes to a daily diet. 2,000 calories a day is used for general nutrition advice.

2 CHO + 0 PRO + 0 FAT

20 oz (600 ml) water

1 tbsp (15 g) honey, amber, organic

4 tsp (20 g) sugar, white, granulated

1/8 tsp (0.6 g) table salt

2 tsp (10 ml) lemon juice, bottled

Heat 1 cup of water in a microwave. Add the hot water to a pitcher, and dissolve the honey, sugar, and salt. Add the lemon juice and remaining water. Pour into a 20-ounce (600 ml) bottle and chill.

Nutrition Facts

1 serving per container

Serving size   20 ounce bottle (616g)

Amount per serving

Calories 140

% Daily Value*

Total Fat 0g	**0%**
Saturated Fat 0g	**0%**
Trans Fat 0g	
Cholesterol 0mg	**0%**
Sodium 320mg	**13%**
Total Carbohydrate 34g	**11%**
Dietary Fiber 0g	**0%**
Total Sugars 33g	
Includes 33g Added Sugars	
Protein 0g	
Vitamin D 0mcg	0%
Calcium 18mg	2%
Iron 0mg	0%
Potassium 11mg	0%

* The % Daily Value (DV) tells you how much a nutrient in a serving of food contributes to a daily diet. 2,000 calories a day is used for general nutrition advice.

Sport Drink 3

2 CHO + 0 PRO + 0 FAT

14 oz (420 ml) water

6 oz (180 ml) juice (cranberry, pomegranate, cherry blend)

1/10 tsp (0.5 g) table salt

2 tsp (10 g) sugar, white, granulated

Heat 1 cup of water in a microwave. Add the hot water to a pitcher, and dissolve the sugar and salt. Add the juice and remaining water. Pour into a 20-ounce (600 ml) bottle and chill.

Nutrition Facts

1 serving per container

Serving size 20 ounce bottle (576g)

Amount per serving

Calories 130

	% Daily Value*
Total Fat 0g	0%
Saturated Fat 0g	0%
Trans Fat 0g	
Cholesterol 0mg	0%
Sodium 270mg	11%
Total Carbohydrate 32g	11%
Dietary Fiber 0g	0%
Total Sugars 32g	
Includes 32g Added Sugars	
Protein 0g	
Vitamin D 0mcg	0%
Calcium 12mg	2%
Iron 0mg	0%
Potassium 0mg	0%

* The % Daily Value (DV) tells you how much a nutrient in a serving of food contributes to a daily diet. 2,000 calories a day is used for general nutrition advice.

Sport Drink 4

2 CHO + 0 PRO + 0 FAT

8 oz (240 ml) coconut water, natural

12 oz (360 ml) water

1/10 tsp (0.5 g) table salt

4 tsp (20 g) sugar, white, granulated

Heat 4 ounces (120 ml) of water in a microwave. Add the hot water to a pitcher, and dissolve the sugar and salt. Add coconut water and the remaining water. Pour into a 20-ounce (600 ml) bottle and chill.

Nutrition Facts

1 serving per container

Serving size 20 ounce bottle (584g)

Amount per serving

Calories 110

	% Daily Value*
Total Fat 0g	0%
Saturated Fat 0g	0%
Trans Fat 0g	
Cholesterol 0mg	0%
Sodium 290mg	12%
Total Carbohydrate 27g	9%
Dietary Fiber 0g	0%
Total Sugars 26g	
Includes 26g Added Sugars	
Protein 0g	
Vitamin D 0mcg	0%
Calcium 38mg	4%
Iron 0mg	0%
Potassium 459mg	10%

* The % Daily Value (DV) tells you how much a nutrient in a serving of food contributes to a daily diet. 2,000 calories a day is used for general nutrition advice.

Sport Drink 5 (3 Quarts)

2 CHO + 0 PRO + 0 FAT

11 cups water

3/4 cup sugar, white, granulated

1/2 tsp (2.5 g) table salt

5 tbsp (75 ml) lime juice

Dissolve the salt and sugar in 3 cups of warm water. Once it is completely dissolved, add it to the remaining water. Add the lime juice. Mix well.

Nutrition Facts

12 servings per container

Serving size 8 ounces (236g)

Amount per serving

Calories 50

% Daily Value*

Total Fat 0g	**0%**
Saturated Fat 0g	**0%**
Trans Fat 0g	
Cholesterol 0mg	**0%**
Sodium 105mg	**4%**
Total Carbohydrate 13g	**4%**
Dietary Fiber 0g	
Total Sugars 13g	
Includes 13g Added Sugars	
Protein 0g	
Vitamin D 0mcg	0%
Calcium 7mg	0%
Iron 0mg	0%
Potassium 6mg	0%

* The % Daily Value (DV) tells you how much a nutrient in a serving of food contributes to a daily diet. 2,000 calories a day is used for general nutrition advice.

Chapter 11

Solid-Fuel Recipes

This chapter provides ideas and recipes for solid, easily digested fueling options such as energy bars and a variety of high-protein selections.

Energy Bars

Many parents and athletes want to know the best nutrition or energy bar to take to school or eat after exercise. What's best depends on what you are using it for. Are you eating it as your breakfast? Is it to satisfy hunger after school? Are you looking for a preworkout bar, or do you need something convenient for immediately after activity?

Bars with high carbohydrate receive a lot of negative press, but a bar with quick-digesting carbohydrate, low fiber and fat, and just a bit of protein is what a cyclist on a long-distance ride really needs. It can also be a good option for a swimmer who has to fuel up before the next event. That same bar, however, would not be the best choice as you are running out of the house for school. A good bar for breakfast includes complex carbohydrate, fiber, protein, and even a little fat.

A bar to have after activity should contain a balance of nutrients, but the size depends on how exhaustive the exercise was. After an hour-long training session, a smaller 150- to 200-calorie balanced bar might be enough; for athletes with high calorie needs, a 300- to 400-calorie bar might be more appropriate.

Because I get so many questions about the best bar, I want to address how different bars fit into the meal plan. And because not many bars have the balance of high-quality nutrients I want, I share how you can make them as well as how they will fit into your meal plan. This way you can also compare their nutrition facts and ingredients lists to those of other bars on the market. I purposely use a lot of the same ingredients in these recipes so that you can have them on hand.

Balanced Breakfast Bar

2 CHO + 1 PRO + 2 FAT

1 tsp (5 g) cinnamon

1/3 cup brown rice syrup

1 tsp (5 ml) vanilla extract

1/3 cup almond butter

1/4 cup almonds, whole, unsalted, chopped

1/4 cup tropical fruit, dried, chopped

1 cup crispy rice cereal

1 cup oats, old-fashioned

1 1/2 scoops (32 g) whey protein powder, vanilla

1/8 tsp (0.6 g) table salt

Nutrition Facts
8 servings per container

Serving size	**1 bar (52g)**

Amount per serving	
Calories	**220**

	% Daily Value*
Total Fat 9g	**14%**
Saturated Fat 1g	**5%**
Trans Fat 0g	
Cholesterol 10mg	**3%**
Sodium 110mg	**5%**
Total Carbohydrate 28g	**9%**
Dietary Fiber 3g	**12%**
Total Sugars 11g	
Includes 7g Added Sugars	
Protein 8g	
Vitamin D 0mcg	0%
Calcium 76mg	8%
Iron 2mg	10%
Potassium 184mg	4%

* The % Daily Value (DV) tells you how much a nutrient in a serving of food contributes to a daily diet. 2,000 calories a day is used for general nutrition advice.

Preheat oven to 300 °F (150 °C). Line an 8- by 8-inch (20 by 20 cm) pan with parchment paper. Cut the paper long enough so that it hangs over the sides.

Combine rice cereal, oats, protein powder, cinnamon, salt, and chopped almonds in a large bowl. Mix well and set aside.

Place the brown rice syrup, vanilla, almond butter, and diced fruit pieces in a microwavable bowl and microwave for 30 seconds on high. Stir with a spoon until evenly blended.

Add the liquid ingredients to the dry ingredients, and use a sturdy spoon to mix. Using a bit of cooking spray on the spoon will help prevent sticking. You can also use your hands to stir. Mix well so that everything is moist.

Once it is mixed, spread evenly into the pan. Use another piece of parchment paper to press the mixture firmly and evenly into the pan using a heavy steel spatula. If the mixture isn't pressed firmly enough, the bar will crumble after cooking. Press firmly around the edges and all areas of the pan. Once it is pressed, remove the parchment paper you used to press. The mixture should appear tight, flat, and even in the pan.

Bake for 20 minutes. Remove the pan from the oven and let it cool. Once cooled, refrigerate for one to two hours, remove from the pan, and cut into eight bars. Refrigerate or freeze.

Preworkout Energy Bar

Recipe developed by Sara Hass, RDN, LDN

1.5 CHO + 0.5 PRO + 1 FAT

1 1/2 cups oats, old-fashioned

1/4 cup peanuts, dry roasted, unsalted, chopped

1 tsp (5 g) cinnamon

1/4 tsp (1.3 g) table salt

1/4 cup peanut butter, creamy

1/3 cup honey, amber

1/3 cup cranberries, dried, sweetened

1/2 tsp (2.5 g) vanilla extract

Nutrition Facts	
12 servings per container	
Serving size	**1 bar (32g)**
Amount per serving	
Calories	**130**
	% Daily Value*
Total Fat 5g	8%
Saturated Fat 1g	5%
Trans Fat 0g	
Cholesterol 0mg	0%
Sodium 75mg	3%
Total Carbohydrate 19g	6%
Dietary Fiber 2g	8%
Total Sugars 10g	
Includes 7g Added Sugars	
Protein 3g	
Vitamin D 0mcg	0%
Calcium 4mg	0%
Iron 0.7mg	4%
Potassium 0mg	0%

* The % Daily Value (DV) tells you how much a nutrient in a serving of food contributes to a daily diet. 2,000 calories a day is used for general nutrition advice.

Preheat oven to 300 °F (150 °C). Line an 8- by 8-inch (20 by 20 cm) pan with two pieces of parchment paper so they are overlapping in the pan and cut long enough to allow some overhang.

Mix the oats, chopped peanuts, cinnamon, and salt together in a large bowl and set aside.

In a microwavable measuring cup, combine the peanut butter, honey, fruit, and vanilla. Cover and microwave for 35 seconds on high. Stir, then pour the peanut butter mixture over the oat mixture and stir to combine until the oats are well coated. Spread the mixture evenly into the prepared pan. Use another piece of parchment paper to press the mixture firmly into the pan with a heavy steel spatula. Press firmly around the edges and all areas of the pan. If the mixture isn't pressed firmly enough, the bar will crumble after cooking. Once it is pressed, remove the parchment paper used to press. The mixture should appear tight, flat, and even in the pan.

Bake for 15 minutes. Remove from the oven and let it cool. Once cooled, refrigerate for one to two hours, remove from the pan, and cut into 12 bars. Refrigerate or freeze.

High-Calorie Preworkout Energy Bar

Recipe developed by Sara Hass, RDN, LDN

2.5 CHO + 1 PRO + 2 FAT

1 1/2 cups oats, old-fashioned

1/4 cup peanuts, dry roasted, unsalted, chopped

1 tsp (5 g) cinnamon

1/4 tsp (1.3 g) table salt

1/4 cup peanut butter, creamy

1/3 cup honey, amber

1/3 cup cranberries, dried, sweetened

1/2 tsp (2.5 g) vanilla extract

Nutrition Facts	
6 servings per container	
Serving size	**1 bar (63g)**

Amount per serving	
Calories	**260**

	% Daily Value*
Total Fat 10g	**15%**
Saturated Fat 1.5g	**8%**
Trans Fat 0g	
Cholesterol 0mg	**0%**
Sodium 150mg	**6%**
Total Carbohydrate 38g	**13%**
Dietary Fiber 3g	**12%**
Total Sugars 20g	
Includes 14g Added Sugars	
Protein 7g	
Vitamin D 0mcg	0%
Calcium 0mg	0%
Iron 1.3mg	8%
Potassium 0mg	0%

* The % Daily Value (DV) tells you how much a nutrient in a serving of food contributes to a daily diet. 2,000 calories a day is used for general nutrition advice.

Preheat oven to 300 °F (150 °C). Line an 8- by 8-inch (20 by 20 cm) pan with two pieces of parchment paper so they are overlapping in the pan and cut long enough to allow some overhang.

Mix the oats, chopped peanuts, cinnamon, and salt together in a large bowl and set aside.

In a microwavable measuring cup, combine the peanut butter, honey, fruit, and vanilla. Cover and microwave for 35 seconds on high. Stir, then pour the peanut butter mixture over the oat mixture and stir to combine, until the oats are well coated. Spread the mixture evenly into the prepared pan. Use another piece of parchment paper to press the mixture firmly into the pan with a heavy steel spatula. Press firmly around the edges and all areas of the pan. If the mixture isn't pressed firmly enough, the bar will crumble after cooking. Once it is pressed, remove the parchment paper used to press. The mixture should appear tight, flat, and even in the pan.

Bake for 15 minutes. Remove from the oven and let it cool. Once cooled, refrigerate for one to two hours, remove from the pan, and cut into six bars. Refrigerate or freeze.

Recipe developed by Sara Hass, RDN, LDN

1.5 CHO + 1 PRO + 2 FAT

1 cup oats, old-fashioned

1/4 tsp (1.3 g) table salt

6 tbsp (90 g) hemp seeds

1/2 cup wheat germ

1/3 cup peanuts, dry roasted, unsalted, chopped

1/3 cup almonds, whole, unsalted, chopped

1/2 tsp (2.5 g) cinnamon

1/2 cup prunes

1/2 cup raisins, seedless

1/4 cup peanut butter, creamy

2 tbsp (30 ml) maple syrup

1 tbsp (15 g) honey, amber

Nutrition Facts

12 servings per container

Serving size	1 bar (49g)

Amount per serving

Calories **210**

	% Daily Value*
Total Fat 10g	**15%**
Saturated Fat 1g	**5%**
Trans Fat 0g	
Cholesterol 0mg	**0%**
Sodium 70mg	**3%**
Total Carbohydrate 24g	**8%**
Dietary Fiber 4g	**16%**
Total Sugars 13g	
Includes 3.5g Added Sugars	
Protein 7g	
Vitamin D 0mcg	0%
Calcium 27mg	2%
Iron 1.8mg	10%
Potassium 167mg	4%

* The % Daily Value (DV) tells you how much a nutrient in a serving of food contributes to a daily diet. 2,000 calories a day is used for general nutrition advice.

Preheat oven to 300 °F (150 °C). Line an 8- by 8-inch (20 by 20 cm) pan with two pieces of parchment paper so they are overlapping in the pan and cut long enough to allow some over-hang.

Mix the oats, hemp seeds, wheat germ, cinnamon, salt, chopped peanuts, and chopped almonds together in a large bowl and set aside.

Place prunes and raisins in a food processor and pulse until very finely chopped. The mixture will begin to clump and form a paste. Add the fruit to the dry ingredients, using a sturdy spoon to mix. Spraying a bit of cooking spray on the spoon will help prevent sticking. You can also use your hands to stir. Mix well so that everything is moist.

In a microwavable measuring cup, combine the peanut butter, honey, and maple syrup. Cover and microwave for 30 seconds on medium heat. Stir, then pour the peanut butter mixture over the oat mixture. Using a sturdy spoon, stir to combine. Once well mixed (everything should appear moist), spread the mixture evenly into the prepared pan. Use another piece of parchment paper to press the mixture firmly into the pan with a heavy steel spatula. Press firmly around the edges and all areas of the pan. If the mixture isn't pressed firmly enough, the bar will crumble after cooking. Once it is pressed, remove the parchment paper used to press. The mixture should appear tight, flat, and even in the pan.

Bake for 15 minutes. Remove from the oven and let it cool. Once cooled, refrigerate for one to two hours, remove from the pan, and cut into 12 bars. Refrigerate or freeze.

High-Calorie Postworkout Energy Bar

3 CHO + 2 PRO + 3 FAT

2 cups oats, old-fashioned

3/4 cup hemp seeds

1 cup wheat germ

1 tsp (5 g) cinnamon

2/3 cup peanuts, dry roasted, unsalted, chopped

2/3 cup almonds, whole, unsalted, chopped

1 cup prunes

1 cup raisins, seedless

1/2 cup peanut butter, creamy

4 tbsp (60 g) light honey

4 tbsp (60 ml) maple syrup

1/2 tsp (2.5 g) table salt

Nutrition Facts	
14 servings per container	
Serving size	**1 bar (87g)**
Amount per serving	
Calories	**360**
	% Daily Value*
Total Fat 17g	**26%**
Saturated Fat 2g	**10%**
Trans Fat 0g	
Cholesterol 0mg	**0%**
Sodium 130mg	**5%**
Total Carbohydrate 44g	**15%**
Dietary Fiber 6g	**24%**
Total Sugars 24g	
Includes 8g Added Sugars	
Protein 13g	
Vitamin D 0mcg	0%
Calcium 45mg	4%
Iron 3mg	20%
Potassium 290mg	6%

* The % Daily Value (DV) tells you how much a nutrient in a serving of food contributes to a daily diet. 2,000 calories a day is used for general nutrition advice.

Preheat oven to 300 °F (150 °C). Line a 9- by 13-inch (23 by 33 cm) pan with two pieces of parchment paper so they are overlapping in the pan and cut long enough to allow some overhang.

Mix the oats, hemp seeds, wheat germ, cinnamon, salt, chopped peanuts, and chopped almonds together in a large bowl and set aside.

Place prunes and raisins in a food processor and pulse until very finely chopped. The mixture will begin to clump and form a paste. Add the fruit to the dry ingredients, using a sturdy spoon to mix. Spraying a bit of cooking spray on the spoon will help prevent sticking. You can also use your hands to stir. Mix well so that everything is moist.

In a microwavable measuring cup, combine the peanut butter, honey, and maple syrup. Cover and microwave for 30 seconds on medium heat. Stir, then pour the peanut butter mixture over the oat mixture. Using a sturdy spoon, stir to combine. Once well mixed (everything should appear moist), spread the mixture evenly into the prepared pan. Use another piece of parchment paper to press the mixture firmly into the pan with a heavy steel spatula. Press firmly around the edges and all areas of the pan. If the mixture isn't pressed firmly enough, the bar will crumble after cooking. Once it is pressed, remove the parchment paper used to press. The mixture should appear tight, flat, and even in the pan.

Bake for 15 minutes. Remove from the oven and let it cool. Once cooled, refrigerate for one to two hours, remove from the pan, and cut into 14 bars. Refrigerate or freeze.

Gluten-Free Energy Bar

Recipe developed by Sara Hass, RDN, LDN

1 CHO + 0 PRO + 1 FAT

1 cup almonds, whole, unsalted

1/4 cup coconut, dried, unsweetened

1/3 cup pineapple, dried

1/2 cup crispy rice cereal

1/4 tsp (1.3 g) table salt

1/4 cup honey, amber

1/2 tsp (2.5 g) vanilla extract

Nutrition Facts	
12 servings per container	
Serving size	**1 bar (25g)**
Amount per serving	
Calories	**120**
	% Daily Value*
Total Fat 7g	**11%**
Saturated Fat 1.5g	**8%**
Trans Fat 0g	
Cholesterol 0mg	**0%**
Sodium 55mg	**2%**
Total Carbohydrate 12g	**4%**
Dietary Fiber 2g	**8%**
Total Sugars 9g	
Includes 5g Added Sugars	
Protein 3g	
Vitamin D 0mcg	0%
Calcium 34mg	4%
Iron 0.8mg	4%
Potassium 106mg	2%

* The % Daily Value (DV) tells you how much a nutrient in a serving of food contributes to a daily diet. 2,000 calories a day is used for general nutrition advice.

Preheat oven to 350 °F (180 °C). Line an 8- by 8-inch (20 by 20 cm) pan with two pieces of parchment paper so they are overlapping in the pan and cut long enough to allow some overhang.

Combine almonds, coconut, pineapple, cereal, and salt in a large mixing bowl. Set aside.

In a microwavable measuring cup, combine the honey and vanilla. Cover and microwave for 30 seconds on high. Stir, then pour the honey and vanilla over the dry mixture. Using a sturdy spoon, stir to combine. Once well mixed (everything should appear moist), spread the mixture evenly into the prepared pan. Use another piece of parchment paper to press the mixture firmly into the pan with a heavy steel spatula. Press firmly around the edges and all areas of the pan. If the mixture isn't pressed firmly enough, the bar will crumble after cooking. Once it is pressed, remove the parchment paper used to press. The mixture should appear tight, flat, and even in the pan.

Bake for 15 minutes. Remove from the oven and let it cool. Once cooled, refrigerate for one to two hours, remove from the pan, and cut into 12 bars. Refrigerate or freeze.

Simple Fruit and Nut Bar

2.5 CHO + 0.5 PRO + 2 FAT

1 cup cashew halves, roasted and salted

32 dates, whole

Line an 8- by 8-inch (20 by 20 cm) pan with two pieces of parchment paper so they are overlapping in the pan and cut long enough to allow some overhang.

Place the cashews in a food processor and chop until finely chopped, but not pastelike. Place them in a bowl and set aside. Add the dates to the food processor and blend until pastelike. Add the cashews and pulse until the ingredients are well blended.

Spread the mixture evenly into the prepared pan. Use another piece of parchment paper to press the mixture firmly into the pan. If necessary, use a spatula or other utensil to help press the mixture firmly. Once it is pressed, remove the parchment paper used to press. The mixture should appear tight, flat, and even in the pan.

Refrigerate for 30 minutes and cut into six bars. Wrap each bar in plastic wrap and store them in the refrigerator.

Nutrition Facts

6 servings per container

Serving size 1 bar (60g)

Amount per serving

Calories 240

	% Daily Value*
Total Fat 10g	**15%**
Saturated Fat 2g	**10%**
Trans Fat 0g	
Cholesterol 0mg	**0%**
Sodium 65mg	**3%**
Total Carbohydrate 38g	**13%**
Dietary Fiber 4g	**16%**
Total Sugars 29g	
Includes 0g Added Sugars	
Protein 5g	
Vitamin D 0mcg	0%
Calcium 30mg	2%
Iron 1.65mg	10%
Potassium 136mg	3%

* The % Daily Value (DV) tells you how much a nutrient in a serving of food contributes to a daily diet. 2,000 calories a day is used for general nutrition advice.

Fruit, Nut, and Chocolate Energy Bar

1.5 CHO + 1 PRO + 2.5 FAT

1 cup peanuts, dry roasted, unsalted

15 dates

2 tbsp (30 g) chocolate chips, semisweet

Line an 8- by 8-inch (20 by 20 cm) pan with two pieces of parchment paper so they are overlapping in the pan and cut long enough to allow some overhang.

Place the chocolate chips in a food processor and chop lightly. Place them in a bowl and set aside. Place the peanuts in the food processor and chop finely. Add them to the bowl. Place the dates in the food processor and blend until pastelike. Add them to the bowl and mix all the ingredients together, blending well.

Spread the mixture evenly into the prepared pan. Use another piece of parchment paper to press the mixture firmly into the pan with a heavy steel spatula. Press firmly around the edges and all areas of the pan. If the mixture isn't pressed firmly enough, the bar can fall apart after cooking. Once it is pressed, remove the parchment paper used to press. The mixture should appear tight, flat, and even in the pan.

Cut into six bars. Wrap each bar in plastic wrap and store them in the refrigerator.

Nutrition Facts

6 servings per container

Serving size   **1 bar (47g)**

Amount per serving

Calories 220

% Daily Value*

Total Fat 13g	**20%**
Saturated Fat 2.5g	**13%**
Trans Fat 0g	
Cholesterol 0mg	**0%**
Sodium 0mg	**0%**
Total Carbohydrate 23g	**8%**
Dietary Fiber 4g	**16%**
Total Sugars 17g	
Includes 3g Added Sugars	
Protein 7g	
Vitamin D 0mcg	0%
Calcium 29mg	2%
Iron 1.65mg	4%
Potassium 136mg	3%

* The % Daily Value (DV) tells you how much a nutrient in a serving of food contributes to a daily diet. 2,000 calories a day is used for general nutrition advice.

Portable Protein

Finding food to eat quickly on the go is not necessarily the hard part; finding the right balance of nutrients can be. In my experience, the biggest barrier is finding portable protein choices that can be made in advance and consumed quickly. As noted in chapter 9, meal preparation should be quick and easy. You don't need fancy ingredients to put together a healthy meal. Each of the following recipes provides at least one portion of protein and can be prepped in advance and stored in the refrigerator for the entire week.

Trail Mix

2 CHO + 1 PRO + 1 FAT

1/4 cup chocolate chips, mini, semisweet

1/2 cup cranberries, dried, sweetened

1/2 cup soybeans, dry roasted, mature

2 oz (60 g) pretzel nuggets, multigrain with sesame seeds

Mix all ingredients evenly in a large plastic bag. Scoop six individual half-cup portions into small plastic bags.

Nutrition Facts	
6 servings per container	
Serving size	**1/2 cup (46g)**
Amount per serving	
Calories	**190**
	% Daily Value*
Total Fat 6g	**9%**
Saturated Fat 2g	**10%**
Trans Fat 0g	
Cholesterol 0mg	**0%**
Sodium 95mg	**4%**
Total Carbohydrate 30g	**10%**
Dietary Fiber 3g	**12%**
Total Sugars 11g	
Includes 4g Added Sugars	
Protein 8g	
Vitamin D 0.11mcg	1%
Calcium 35mg	4%
Iron 3mg	15%
Potassium 245mg	5%

* The % Daily Value (DV) tells you how much a nutrient in a serving of food contributes to a daily diet. 2,000 calories a day is used for general nutrition advice.

Protein-Rich Overnight Oats

2 CHO + 1 PRO + 0 FAT

3 cups oats, old-fashioned

2 tbsp (60 g) wheat germ

10 strawberries, medium

2 bananas, medium

2 tbsp (60 g) honey, amber

4 cups milk, skim, with vitamins A and D

1/2 cup hot water

Combine the oats and wheat germ in a large bowl and set aside.

Place the strawberries and bananas into a food processor and puree until smooth (if using frozen fruit, add 1/2 cup hot water). Add the fruit mixture, milk, and syrup to the dry ingredients and mix well. Cover and store in the refrigerator overnight. In the morning, add the amount you want to eat to a bowl, heat in microwave or on the stove top, and eat. It will keep in the refrigerator for up to five days.

Nutrition Facts	
10 servings per container	
Serving size	**3/4 cup (182g)**

Amount per serving	
Calories	**170**

	% Daily Value*
Total Fat 2g	**3%**
Saturated Fat 0g	**0%**
Trans Fat 0g	
Cholesterol 0mg	**0%**
Sodium 40mg	**2%**
Total Carbohydrate 32g	**11%**
Dietary Fiber 4g	**16%**
Total Sugars 13g	
Includes 3g Added Sugars	
Protein 7g	
Vitamin D 1.2mcg	1%
Calcium 124mg	10%
Iron 1.3mg	8%
Potassium 259mg	6%

* The % Daily Value (DV) tells you how much a nutrient in a serving of food contributes to a daily diet. 2,000 calories a day is used for general nutrition advice.

Cottage Cheese Pancakes

0.5 CHO + 1 PRO + 0.5 FAT

2 eggs, large

1 cup cottage cheese, 2%

1 cup oats, old-fashioned

4 egg whites, large

1 tsp (5 g) baking powder

1 tsp (5 ml) vanilla extract

1/8 tsp (0.6 g) cinnamon

Place the cottage cheese in a food processor and blend until smooth. Place it in a bowl and set aside.

Place the oats in a food processor and blend to make oat flour. Add to the cottage cheese and stir well. Add all the other ingredients.

Use a 1/2 cup measuring cup to portion the batter into pancakes on a hot griddle.

Nutrition Facts	
11 servings per container	
Serving size 1 pancake (55g)	

Amount per serving

Calories	**70**

	% Daily Value*
Total Fat 2g	3%
Saturated Fat 0.5g	3%
Trans Fat 0g	
Cholesterol 45mg	15%
Sodium 150mg	6%
Total Carbohydrate 7g	2%
Dietary Fiber 1g	4%
Total Sugars 1g	
Includes 0g Added Sugars	
Protein 7g	
Vitamin D 0mcg	0%
Calcium 64mg	6%
Iron 0.6mg	4%
Potassium 41mg	1%

* The % Daily Value (DV) tells you how much a nutrient in a serving of food contributes to a daily diet. 2,000 calories a day is used for general nutrition advice.

Egg Muffins

O CHO + 1 PRO + 1 FAT

18 eggs, large

6 egg whites, large

1/2 cup onion, white, chopped

1/4 tsp (1.3 g) table salt

1/8 tsp (0.6 g) black pepper

6 sausage links, turkey, precooked, frozen

1 cup baby spinach

10 cherry tomatoes

Preheat oven to 350 °F (180 °C). Spray a muffin tin with cooking spray. Crack all the eggs and egg whites and beat them together in a large bowl. Set aside.

In a food processor, chop the onion and sausage into crumbled pieces. Add them to the egg mixture. Using a sharp knife, chop the spinach and cut the tomatoes into small pieces and add them to the egg mixture. Add salt and pepper and mix well.

Fill each muffin tin three-quarters full (should be enough to fill 24 tins). Bake for 20 to 25 minutes, or until a food thermometer reads 160 °F (70 °C).

Nutrition Facts

24 servings per container

Serving size   **1 muffin (62g)**

Amount per serving

Calories   70

% Daily Value*

Total Fat 4g	**6%**
Saturated Fat 1.5g	**8%**
Trans Fat 0g	
Cholesterol 165mg	**55%**
Sodium 125mg	**5%**
Total Carbohydrate 2g	**1%**
Dietary Fiber 0g	**0%**
Total Sugars 0g	
Includes 0g Added Sugars	
Protein 6g	
Vitamin D 0mcg	0%
Calcium 23mg	2%
Iron 0.7mg	4%
Potassium 35mg	1%

* The % Daily Value (DV) tells you how much a nutrient in a serving of food contributes to a daily diet. 2,000 calories a day is used for general nutrition advice.

Basic Turkey Meatballs

0 CHO + 1 PRO + 0.5 FAT

2 lb (1 kg) turkey, ground, 7% fat

2 eggs, large

1/2 cup bread crumbs, plain

1/4 tsp (1.3 g) black pepper

Preheat oven to 350 °F (180 °C). Spray a 9- by 13-inch (23 by 33 cm) baking dish with cooking spray.

Mix all ingredients together in a large bowl using your hands. Form the meat mixture into 1.5-ounce (45 g) balls and place them in the baking dish.

Bake uncovered for 25 minutes. Serve plain or with pasta sauce. Store unused meatballs in the freezer.

Nutrition Facts

27 servings per container

Serving size 1 meatball (39g)

Amount per serving

Calories 60

	% Daily Value*
Total Fat 2.5g	4%
Saturated Fat 0.5g	3%
Trans Fat 0g	
Cholesterol 35mg	12%
Sodium 45mg	2%
Total Carbohydrate 1g	0%
Dietary Fiber 0g	0%
Total Sugars 0g	
Includes 0g Added Sugars	
Protein 7g	
Vitamin D 0mcg	0%
Calcium 5mg	0%
Iron 0.7mg	4%
Potassium 0mg	0%

* The % Daily Value (DV) tells you how much a nutrient in a serving of food contributes to a daily diet. 2,000 calories a day is used for general nutrition advice.

Bibliography

Accuracy Research LLP. 2016. Global Sports nutrition and supplements market analysis & trends: Industry forecast to 2020. Research and Markets. www.researchandmarkets.com/research/z3bh86/global_sports.

Adams, J.D., Kavouras, S.A., Robillard, J.I., et al. 2016. Fluid balance of adolescent swimmers during training. *Journal of Strength and Conditioning Research* 30 (3): 621-625.

Aegis Sciences Corporation. www.aegislabs.com.

American Academy of Child & Adolescent Psychiatry. 2011, December. Normal adolescent development part I. Facts for Families Guide, No. 57. https://www.aacap.org/App_Themes/AACAP/docs/facts_for_families /57_normal_adolescent_development.pdf.

American Academy of Child and Adolescent Psychiatry. 2011, December. Normal adolescent development part II. Facts for Families Guide, No. 58. http://www.aacap.org/AACAP/Families_and_Youth/Facts_for_Families/FFF-Guide/Normal-Adolescent-Development-Part-II-058. aspx.

American Academy of Child & Adolescent Psychiatry. 2011, December. Teen brain: Behavior, problem solving, and decision making. Facts for Families Guide, No. 95. http://www.aacap.org/AACAP/Families_and_Youth/ Facts_for_Families/FFF-Guide/The-Teen-Brain-Behavior-Problem-Solving-and-Decision-Making-095.aspx.

American Academy of Pediatrics. 2005. Promotion of healthy weight-control practices in youth athletes. *Pediatrics* 116 (6): 1557-1564.

American College of Sports Medicine, Academy of Nutrition and Dietetics, and Dietitians of Canada. 2016. Joint position statement. Nutrition and athletic performance. March 2016. Vol 1(16-93).

American College of Sports Medicine. 2007. Position stand paper: Exercise and fluid replacement. Medicine & Science in Sports Exercise. 377-389.

American Psychiatric Association. 2013. *Diagnostic and Statistical Manual of Mental Disorders, fifth edition (DSM-5)*. Washington D.C. American Psychiatric Association.

Aragon, A.A., and Schoenfeld, B.J. 2013. Nutrient timing revisited: Is there a post-exercise anabolic window. *Journal of the International Society of Sports Nutrition* 10 (1): 5.

Arciero, Paul, et al. 2015. Performance enhancing diets and the PRISE protocol to optimize athletic performance. *Journal of Nutrition and Metabolism* 2015: 715859.

Arnaoutis, G., Kavouras, S.A., Angelopoulou, A., et al. 2015. Fluid balance during training in elite young athletes of different sports. *Journal of Strength and Conditioning Research* 29 (12): 3447-3452.

Bailes, J.E., and Patel, V. 2014. The potential for DHA to mitigate mild traumatic brain injury. *Military Medicine* 179 (11 Suppl.): 112-116.

Bailey, S.J. 2009. Dietary nitrate supplementation reduces the O2 cost of low-intensity exercise and enhances tolerance to high-intensity exercise in humans. *Journal of Applied Physiology* 107 (4): 1144-1155.

Baker, L.B., Heaton, L.E., Nuccio, R.P., et al. 2014. Dietitian-observed macronutrient intake of young skill and team-sport athletes: Adequacy of pre, during and post exercise nutrition. *International Journal of Sport Nutrition and Exercise Metabolism* 24 (2): 166-176.

Balsom, P.D., et al. 1994. Creatine in humans with special reference to creatine supplementation. *Sports Medicine* 18 (4): 268-280.

Banned Substance Control Group. www.bscg.org.

Bar-Or, Oded. 2001. Nutritional considerations of the child athlete. *Canadian Journal of Applied Physiology* 26 (Suppl.): S186-S191.

Bell, Pg, et al. 2014. The role of cherries in exercise and health. *Scandinavian Journal of Medicine & Science in Sports* 24 (3): 477-490.

Bellinger, P.M. 2014. B-alanine supplementation for athletic performance: An update. *Journal of Strength and Conditioning Research* 28 (6): 1751-1770.

Berenbaum, S.A., Beltz, A.M., and Corley R. 2015. The Importance of puberty for adolescent development: Conceptualization and measurement. *Advances in Child Development and Behavior* 48: 53-92.

Bex, Tine, et al. 2015. Exercise training and beta-alanine induced muscle carnosine loading. *Frontiers in Nutrition* 7: 2:13.

Bloodworth, A.J., et al. 2012. Doping and supplementation: The attitudes of talented young athlete. *Scandinavian Journal of Medicine and Science in Sports* 22 (2): 293-301.

Boisseau, N., Vermorel, M., Rance, M., et al. 2007. Protein requirements in male adolescent soccer players. *European Journal of Applied Physiology* 100 (1): 27-33.

Boisseau, Natalie, Vera-Perez, Sonia, and Poortmans, Jacques. 2005. Food and fluid intake in adolescent female judo athletes before competition. *Pediatric Exercise Science* 17: 62-71.

Bratman, S., and Dunn, Thomas. 2016. On orthorexia nervosa: A review of the literature and proposed diagnostic criteria. *Eating Behaviors* 21: 11-7.

Brennan, Brian, et al. 2010. Human growth hormone abuse in male weightlifters. *American Journal on Addictions* 201 (1): 9-13.

Brown, G.A. 2006. Testosterone prohormone supplements. *Medicine & Science in Sports & Exercise* 38 (8): 1451-1461.

Calfee, Ryan, and Fasdale, Paul. 2006. Popular ergogenic drugs and supplements in young athletes. *Pediatrics* 117: e577-e589.

Carlsohn, Anja, Scharhag-Rosenberger, Friederike, Weber, Josefine, et al. 2011. Physical activity levels to estimate the energy requirement of adolescent athletes. *Pediatric Exercise Science* 23: 261-269.

Casa, D., Armstrong, L., Montain, S., Rich, Brent, et al. 2000. National Athletic Trainers' Association position statement: Fluid replacement for athletes. *Journal of Athletic Training* (2): 212-224.

Center for Science in the Public Interest. https;//cspinet.org.

Chapman, James, and Woodman, Tim. 2016. Disordered eating in male athletes: A meta-analysis. *Journal of Sports Sciences* 34 (2): 101-109.

Choose Your Foods, Academy of Nutrition and Dietetics, 2014. http://www.eatrightstore.org/product/59CD4025-697D-4927-AD71-A8E70D0B1575.

Clarkson, Priscilla, et al. 2000. Antioxidants: What role do they play in physical activity and health? *American Journal of Clinical Nutrition* 72 (Suppl.): 637s-646s.

Cleary, M.A., Hetzler, R.K., Wasson, D., et al. 2012. Hydration behaviors before and after an educational and prescribed hydration intervention in adolescent athletes. *Journal of Athletic Training* 47 (3): 273-281.

Cohen, Pieter, Travis, John, and Venhuis, B.J. 2015. A synthetic stimulant never tested in humans, 1,3 dimethylamylamine (DMAA), is identified in multiple dietary supplements. *Drug Test Analysis* 7: 83-87.

Conolly, D.A.L., et al. 2006. Efficacy of a tart cherry juice blend in preventing the symptoms of muscle damage. *British Journal of Sports Medicine* 40 (8): 679-683.

Consumerlab.org. https://www.consumerlab.com.

Council for Responsible Nutrition (CRN). 2014. The dietary supplement consumer [Survey results]. www.crnusa.org/CRNconsumersurvey/2014/CRN2014CCsurvey-infographic-pages.pdf.

Council for Responsible Nutrition. 2002. Guidelines for young athletes: Responsible use of sports nutrition supplements. http://www.crnusa.org/pdfs/CRNSNSGuidelines1102.pdf.

Council on Sports Medicine and Fitness and Council on School Health, Bergeron, M.F., Devore, C., Rice, S.G., American Academy of Pediatrics. 2011. Policy statement. Climatic heat stress and exercising children and adolescents. *Pediatrics* 128 (3): e741-747.

Deminice, R., et al. 2013. Effects of creatine supplementation on oxidative stress and inflammatory markers after repeated-sprint exercise in humans. *Nutrition* 29 (9): 1127-1132.

Desbrow, Ben, et al. 2009. Caffeine, cycling performance and exogenous CHO oxidation: A dose-response study. *Medicine & Science in Sports & Exercise* 41 (9): 1744-1751.

Deutz, R.C., Benardot, D., Martin, D.E., and Cody, M.M. 2000. Body image concerns, muscle-enhancing behaviors, and eating disorders in males. *Medicine & Science in Sports & Exercise* 32 (3): 659-668.

Deutz, R.C., Benardot, D., Martin, D.E., et al. 2000. Relationship between energy deficits and body composition in elite female gymnasts and runners. *Medicine & Science in Sports & Exercise* 32 (3): 659-668.

Di Santolo, Manuela, Stel, Giuliana, and Banfi, Giuseppe. 2008. Anemia and iron status in young fertile non-professional female athletes. *European Journal of Applied Physiology* 102 (6): 703-709.

Doyle, Daniel. 2013, August. Physical growth and sexual maturation of adolescents: Growth and development. *Merck Manual.* www.merckmanuals.com/home/children-s-health-issues/growth-and-development/physical-growth-and-sexual-maturation-of-adolescents.

Drug Free Sport. www.drugfreesport.com.

Durkalec-Michalski, K., and Jeszka, J. 2016, February 2. The effect of HMB on aerobic capacity and body composition in trained athletes. *Journal of Strength and Conditioning Research.*

Ebbeling, C.B., Swain, J.F., Feldman, H.A., et al. 2012. Effects of dietary composition on energy expenditure during weight-loss maintenance free. *JAMA* 307 (24): 2627-2634.

Eisenburg, Marla, et al. 2012. Muscle-enhancing behaviors among adolescent girls and boys. *Pediatrics* 130 (6): 1019-1026.

Eisenmann, Joey, and Wickel, Eric. 2007. Estimated energy expenditure and physical activity patterns of adolescent distance runners. *International Journal of Sports Nutrition and Exercise Metabolism* 17: 178-188.

Ekelund, Ulf, Ynage, Agneta, Westerterp, Klass, et al. 2002. Energy expenditure assessed by heart rate and doubly labeled water in young athletes. *Medicine & Science in Sports & Exercise* 34 (8): 1360-1366.

Etchison, W.C., Bloodgood, E.A., Minton, C.P., et al. 2011. Body mass index and percentage of body fat as indicators for obesity in an adolescent athletic population. *Sports Health* 3 (3): 249-252.

Eudy, A.E. 2013. Efficacy and safety of ingredients found in preworkout supplements. *American Journal of Health-System Pharmacy* 70 (7): 577-588.

Farrey, Tom. 2010. A legal performance-enhancing drink. ESPN. http://espn.go.com/espn/e60/news/story?id=5726418.

Farzad, Zehsaz., et al. 2014. The effect of *Zingiber officinale R.* rhizomes (ginger) on plasma pro-inflammatory cytokine levels in well-trained male endurance runners. *Central European Journal of Immunology* 39 (2): 174-180.

Fitzgerald, J.S., Peterson, B.J., Warpeha, J.M., Johnson, S.C., and Ingraham, S.J. 2015. Association between vitamin D status and maximal-intensity exercise performance in junior and collegiate hockey players. *Journal of Strength and Conditioning Research* 29 (9): 2513-2521.

Flynn, M.G., MacKinnon, L., Gedge, V., et al. 2003. influence of iron status and iron supplementation on natural killer cell activity in trained women runners. *International Journal of Sports Medicine* 24 (3): 217-222.

Garcia-Cazarin, Mary, et al. 2014. Dietary supplements research portfolio at the NIH, 2009-2011. *Journal of Nutrition* 144 (4): 414-418.

Gerrier, S., and Basiotis, J.W. 2006. An easy approach to calculating estimated energy requirements. *Preventing Chronic Disease* 3 (4): A129.

Giesemer, B.A. 2003. Ergogenic risks elevate health risks in youth athletes. *Pediatric Annals* 32 (11): 733-737.

Gray, P., et al. 2014. Fish oil supplementation reduces markers of oxidative stress but not muscle soreness after eccentric exercise. *International Journal of Sport Nutrition and Exercise Metabolism* 24 (2): 206-214.

Grzanna, R., et al. 2005. Ginger—an herbal medicinal product with broad anti-inflammatory actions. *Journal of Medicinal Food* 8 (2): 125-132.

Hawkins, R.D., Hulse, M.A. Wilkinson, C. Hodson, A., and Gibson, M. 2001. The association football medical research programme: An audit of injuries in professional football. *British Journal of Sports Medicine* 35: 43-47.

Helms, Eric R., et al. 2014. Evidence-based recommendations for natural bodybuilding contest preparation: Nutrition and supplementation. *Journal of the International Society of Sports Nutrition* 11: 20.

Hildebrand, R.A., Miller, B., Warren, A., Hildebrand, D., and Smith, B.J. 2016, April 20. Compromised vitamin d status negatively affects muscular strength and power of collegiate athletes. *International Journal of Sport Nutrition and Exercise Metabolism.*

Hinton, Pamela H., Giordano, Christina, Brownlie, Thomas, et al. 2000. Iron supplementation improves endurance after training in iron-depleted, nonanemic women. *Journal of Applied Physiology* 88 (3): 1103-1111.

Hinton, P.S., and Sinclair, L.M. 2007. Iron supplementation maintains ventilatory threshold and improves energetic efficiency in iron-deficient nonanemic athletes. *European Journal of Clinical Nutrition* 61 (1): 30-39.

Hoffman, Jay, et al. 2008. Nutritional supplementation and anabolic steroid use in adolescents. *Medicine & Science in Sports & Exercise* 40 (1): 15-24.

Hord, Norman, et al. 2008. Food sources of nitrates and nitrites: The physiologic context for potential health benefits. *American Journal of Clinical Nutrition* 90 (1): 1-10.

Hoyte, C.O. 2013. the use of energy drinks, dietary supplements and prescription medications by United States college students to enhance athletic performance. *Journal of Community Health* 38 (3): 575-580.

Hyde, Janet and DeLamater, John. Understanding Human Sexuality. *Sex hormones and sexual Differentiation* Chapter 5. 9th edition. Pages 96-113. McGraw-Hill Education. New York, New York.

Inal, Deniz, et al. 2000. Effects of garlic on aerobic performance. *Turkish Journal of Medical Sciences* 30: 557-561.

Informed-choice.org. http://informed-choice.org.

Ingersoll, G.M. 1992. Psychological and social development. *Textbook of adolescent medicine*, edited by E.R. McAnarney, et al. (Philadelphia: Saunders), 92.

Institute of Medicine. 2010, November. *Dietary reference intakes for calcium and vitamin D*. Washington, DC: National Academies Press.

Ivy, John L., et al. 2009. Improved cycling time-trial performance after ingestion of a caffeine energy drink. *International Journal of Sport Nutrition and Exercise Metabolism* 19 (1): 61-78.

Jeukendrup, A.E. 2010. Carbohydrate and exercise performance: The role of multiple transportable carbohydrates. *Current Opinion in Clinical Nutrition and Metabolic Care* 13 (4): 452-457.

Jeukendrup, A., and Cronin L. 2011. Nutrition and elite young athletes. *Med Sport Sci* 56: 47-58.

Johnson, Sara, Blum, Robert, and Giedd, Jay. 2009. Adolescent maturity and the brain: The promise and pitfalls of neuroscience research in adolescent health policy. *Journal of Adolescent Health* 45 (3): 216-221.

Jones, Andrew, et al. 2014. Dietary nitrate supplementation and exercise performance. *Sports Medicine* 44 (Suppl. 1): S35-S45.

Joy, Elizabeth, De Souza, Mary Jane, Nattiv, Aurelia, et al. 2014. Female athlete triad coalition consensus statement on treatment and return to play of the female athlete triad. *Current Sports Medicine Reports* 13 (4): 219-232.

Judkins, C., et al. 2007. Investigation into supplement contamination levels in the US Market. Survey. www.dopingjouren.se/Global/PDF/Studie_fr-n_HFL.PDF. 1-10.

Juhasz, I., et al. 2009. Creatine supplementation improves the anaerobic performance of elite junior fin swimmers. *Acta Physiologica Hungarica* 96 (3): 325-336.

Karp, J.R., Johnston, J.D., Tecklenburg, S., et al. 2006. Chocolate milk as a post-exercise recovery aid. *International Journal of Sport Nutrition and Exercise Metabolism* 16 (1): 78-91.

Kendall, K.L., et al. 2014. Ingesting a preworkout supplement containing caffeine, creatine, B-alanine, amino acids, and B vitamins for 28 days is both safe and efficacious in recreational active men. *Nutrition Research* 34 (5): 442-449.

Kharirullah, A., Klein, L.C., Ingle, S.M., et al. 2014. Testosterone trajectories and references ranges in a large longitudinal sample of male adolescents. *PLOS ONE* 9 (9): e108838.

Kim, S.Y., Sim, S., and Park, B. 2016. Dietary habits are associated with school performance in adolescents. *Medicine* 95 (12): e3096.

Koo, Ga Hee. 2014. Effects of supplementation with BCAA and L-glutamine on blood fatigue factors and cytokines in juvenile athletes submitted to maximal intensity rowing performance. *Journal of Physical Therapy Science* 26 (8): 1241-1246.

Kong, P., and Harris, L.M. 2015. The sporting body: Body image and eating disorders symptomatology among female athletes from leanness focused and nonleaness focused sports. *Journal of Psychology* 149 (1-2): 141-160.

Kuehl, Kerry, et al. 2010. Efficacy of tart cherry juice in reducing muscle pain during running: A randomized controlled trial. *Journal of the International Society of Sports Nutrition* 7: 17.

Lee, Jae-Seok, et al. 2015. Effects of chronic dietary nitrate supplementation on the hemodynamic response to dynamic exercise. *American Journal of Physiology–Regulatory Integrative and Comparative Physiology* 309 (5): R459-466.

Lewis, Evan J.H., et al. 2105. 21 days of mammalian omega-3 fatty acid supplementation improves aspects of neuromuscular function and performance in male athletes compared to olive oil placebo. *Journal of the International Society of Sports Nutrition* 12: 28.

MacLean, Alice, et al. 2015. "It's not healthy and it's not decidedly not masculine": A media analysis of UK newspaper representations of eating disorders in males. *BMJ Open* 5 (5): e007468.

Mamerow, M., Mettler, J., English, K., et al. 2014. Dietary protein distribution positively influences 24-h muscle protein synthesis in healthy adults. *Journal of Nutrition* 144 (6): 876-880.

Martinsen, Marianne, Bahr, Roald, Borresen, Runi, et al. 2014. Preventing eating disorders among young elite athletes: A randomized controlled trial. *Medicine & Science in Sports & Exercise* 46 (3): 435-447.

Martinsen, Marianne, and Sundgot-Borgen, Jorunn. 2013. Higher prevalence of eating disorders among adolescent athletes than controls. *Medicine & Science in Sports & Exercise* 45 (6): 1188-1197.

Martin- Biggers, J., Spaccarotella, K., Berhaupt-Glickstein, A., et al. 2014. Come and get it! A discussion of family mealtime literature and factors affecting obesity risk. *Advances in Nutrition* 5 (3): 235-247.

Martorell, M., et al. 2014. Effect of DHA on plasma fatty availability and oxidative stress during training season and football exercise. *Food & Function* 5 (8): 1920-1931.

Mashhadi, N.S., et al. 2013. Effect of ginger and cinnamon intake on oxidative stress and exercise performance and body composition in Iranian female athletes. *International Journal of Preventive Medicine* 4 (Suppl. 1): S31-S35.

Matzkin, E., Curry, E.J., and Whitlock, Kaitlyn. 2015. Female athlete triad: Past, present and future. *Journal of the American Academy of Orthopaedic Surgeons* 23 (7): 424-432.

Mayo Clinic. Growth hormone (parenteral route). 2015. www.mayoclinic.org/drugs-supplements/growth-hormone-parenteral-route/side-effects/drg-20069416.

McDowell, Jill Anne. 2007. Supplement use by young athletes. *Journal of Sports Science and Medicine* 6: 337-342.

Evans Jr, Marion Willard, et al. 2012. Dietary supplement use by children and adolescents in the United States to enhance sports performance: Results of the National Health Interview Survey. *Journal of Primary Prevention* 33 (1): 3-12.

McGuine, T.A., Sullivan, J.C., and Bernhardt, D.T. 2001. Creatine supplementation in high school football players. *Clinical Journal of Sports Medicine* 11 (4): 247-253.

Medical Institute for Sexual Health. 2005. Maturation of the teenage brain: Implications for parents, mentors and society. Medical Institute for Sexual Health. Austin, Texas. 2005.

Merkel, Donna L. 2013. Youth sports: A positive and negative impact on young athletes. *Journal of Sports Medicine* 4: 151-160.

Merkel, D., Huerta, M., Grott, I., et al. 2009. Incidence of anemia and iron deficiency in strenuously trained adolescents: Results of a longitudinal follow-up study. *Journal of Adolescent Health* 45 (3): 286-291.

Mettler, S., Mitchell, N., and Tipton, K. 2010. Increased protein intake reduces lean body mass loss during weight loss in athletes. *Medicine & Science in Sports & Exercise* 42 (2): 326-337.

Mickleborough, T.D. 2013. Omega-3 polyunsaturated fatty acids in physical performance optimization. *International Journal of Sport Nutrition and Exercise Metabolism* 23 (1): 83-96.

Milewski, M.D., Skaggs, D.L., Bishop, G.A., et al. 2014. Chronic lack of sleep is associated with increased sports injuries in adolescent athletes. *Journal of Pediatric Orthopedics* 34 (2): 129-133.

Montfort-Steiger, V., and Williams, C.A. 2007. Carbohydrate intake considerations for young athletes. *Journal of Sports Science and Medicine* 6 (3): 343-352.

Moore, D.R., Robinson, M.J., Fry, J.L., et al. 2009. Ingested protein dose response of muscle and albumin protein synthesis after resistance exercise in young men. *American Journal of Clinical Nutrition* 89: 161-168.

Mountjoy, M., Sundgot-Borgen, Jorunn., Burke, L., et al. 2014. The IOC consensus statement: Beyond the female athlete triad—relative energy deficiency in sport (RED-S). *British Journal of Sports Medicine* 48 (7): 491-497.

Mountjoy, M., Sundgot-Borgen, Jorunn, Burke, L., et al. 2015. Authors' 2015 additions to the IOC consensus statement: Relative Energy Deficiency in Sport (RED-S). *British Journal of Sports Medicine* 49 (7): 417-420.

Mountjoy, M., Sundgot-Borgen, Jorunn, Burke, L., et al. 2015. The IOC Relative Energy Deficiency in Sport Clinical Assessment Tool (RED-S CAT). *British Journal of Sports Medicine* 49 (21): 1354.

Mulcahey, M.K., et al. 2010. Anabolic steroid use in adolescents: Identification of those at risk and strategies for prevention. *Physician and Sportsmedicine* 38 (3): 105-113.

Murphy, Margaret, et al. 2012. Whole beetroot consumption acutely improves running performance. *Journal of the Academy of Nutrition and Dietetics* 112 (4): 548-552.

Murray, R., Paul, G.L., Seifert, J.G., et al. 1989. The effects of glucose, fructose and sucrose ingestion during exercise. *Medicine & Science in Sports & Exercise* 21 (3): 275-282.

National Collegiate Athletic Association (NCAA). (n.d.). 2016-17 NCAA banned drugs. www.ncaa.org/2016-17-ncaa-banned-drugs.

National Eating Disorder Association (NEDA). www.nationaleatingdisorders.org.

National Federation of State High School Associations (NFHS), Sports Medicine Advisory Committee (SMAC). 2014. Position statement and recommendations for the use of energy drinks by young athletes. www.nfhs.org/sports-resource-content/position-statement-and-recommendations-for-the-use-of-energy-drinks-by-young-athletes.

National Federation of State High School Associations (NFHS), Sports Medicine Advisory Committee. 2014. Supplements Position Statement. http://www.nfhs.org/sports-resource-content/supplements-position-statement.

National Football League Players Association. 2014. NFL list of prohibited substances. https://nflpaweb.blob.core.windows.net/media/Default/PDFs/Player%20Planner/2014%20NFL%20List%20of%20Prohibited%20Substances.pdf.

National Institutes of Health, Office of Dietary Supplements. 2016. Vitamin D fact sheet. https://ods.od.nih.gov/factsheets/VitaminD-HealthProfessional.

National Institutes of Health, Office of Dietary Supplements. 2016. Calcium fact sheet. https://ods.od.nih.gov/factsheets/Calcium-HealthProfessional.

National Institutes of Health, Office of Dietary Supplements. 2016. Iron fact sheet. https://ods.od.nih.gov/factsheets/Iron-HealthProfessional.

National Sleep Foundation. https://sleepfoundation.org/insomnia/how-sleep-works/why-do-we-need-sleep.

National Sleep Foundation. (n.d.). Sleep drive and your body clock. https://sleepfoundation.org/sleep-topics/sleep-drive-and-your-body-clock.

National Sleep Foundation. (n.d.). Sleep duration recommendations. https://sleepfoundation.org.

Nattiv, A., Loucks, A.B., Manore, M.M., et al. 2007. American College of Sports Medicine position stand: The female athlete triad. *Medicine & Science in Sports and Exercise* 39(10): 1867-1882.

Natural Medicines Comprehensive Database. (n.d.). Echinacea. http://naturaldatabase. therapeuticresearch.com/nd/Search.aspx?cs=&s=ND&pt=100&id=981&fs=ND&search id=57064128.

Natural Medicines Comprehensive Database. (n.d.). Ephedra. http://naturaldatabase.therapeuticresearch.com/nd/Search.aspx?cs=&s=ND&pt=100&id=847&fs=ND&searchid=57064128.

Natural Medicines Comprehensive Database. (n.d.). Garlic. http://naturaldatabase.therapeuticresearch.com/nd/Search.aspx?cs=&s=ND&pt=100&id=300&fs=ND&searchid=57064381.

Natural Medicines Comprehensive Database. (n.d.). Ginger. http://naturaldatabase.therapeuticresearch.com/nd/Search.aspx?cs=&s=ND&pt=100&id=961&fs=ND&searchid=57064241.

Natural Medicines Comprehensive Database. (n.d.). Ginseng, Panax. http://naturaldatabase. therapeuticresearch.com /nd/Search.aspx?cs=&s=nd&pt=100&id=1000.

Natural Medicines Comprehensive Database. (n.d.). Guarana. http://naturaldatabase.therapeuticresearch.com/nd/Search.aspx?cs=&s=ND&pt=100&id=935&fs=ND&searchid=57064128.

Natural Medicines Comprehensive Database. (n.d.). L-carnitine. http://naturaldatabase. therapeuticresearch.com/nd/Search.aspx?cs=&s=ND&pt=100&id=1026&fs=ND&search id=57064128.

Natural Medicines Comprehensive Database. (n.d.). Turmeric. http://naturaldatabase.therapeuticresearch.com/nd/Search.aspx?cs=&s=ND&pt=100&id=662&fs=ND&searchid=57064312.

Nicol, L.M., et al. 2015. Curcumin supplementation likely attenuates delayed onset muscle soreness (DOMS). *European Journal of Applied Physiology* 115 (8): 1769-1777.

Norton, Layne. 2006. Leucine regulates translation initiation of protein synthesis in skeletal muscle after exercise. *Journal of Nutrition* 136 (2): 533S-537S.

NSF Certified for Sport Program. www.nsfsport.com.

Nutrition Business Journal. Supplement business report 2015. 2015. http://newhope.com/sitefiles/newhope360.com/files/uploads/2015/05/2015_SupplementReport_TOC.pdf.

O'Connor, Anahad. 2015. New York attorney general fights to clean up dietary supplement industry. http://well.blogs.nytimes.com/2015/02/03/new-york-attorney-general-targets-supplements-at-major-retailers/?_r=0.

Ogan, Dana, and Pritchett, Kelly. 2013. Vitamin D and the athlete: Risks, recommendations, and benefits. *Nutrients* 5 (6): 1856-1868.

Office of Dietary Supplements. http:ods.od.nih.gov.

Ok Ban, Jung, et al. 2009. Anti-inflammatory and arthritic effects of thiacremonone, a novel sulfur compound isolated from garlic via inhibition of NF-kB. *Arthritis Research & Therapy* 11 (5): R145.

Otten, Jennifer J., Hellwig, Jennifer Pitzi, and Meyers, Linda D., eds. 2006. *DRI, dietary reference intakes: The essential guide to nutrient requirements.* Washington, DC: National Academies Press.

Palmer, M., Logan, H.M., and Lawrence, L. 2010. On-ice sweat rate, voluntary fluid intake, and sodium balance during practice in male junior ice hockey players drinking water or a carbohydrate-electrolyte solution. *Applied Physiology, Nutrition, and Metabolism* 35 (3): 328-335.

Palmer, M., and Spriet, L. 2008. Sweat rate, salt loss, and fluid intake during an intense on-ice practice in elite Canadian male junior hockey players. *Applied Physiology, Nutrition, and Metabolism* 33 (2): 263-271.

Parnell, J.A. 2015. Evaluation of congruence among dietary supplement use and motivation for supplementation in young, Canadian athletes. *Journal of the International Society of Sports Nutrition* Dec 16: 12:49.

Partnership for Drug-Free Kids. 2014. 2013 Partnership Attitude Tracking Study. www.drugfree. org/wp-content/uploads/2014/07/PATS-2013-KEY-FINDINGS1.pdf.

Pasiakos, S.M., Cao, J.J., Margolis, L.M., et al. 2013. Effects of high-protein diets on fat free mass and muscle protein synthesis following weight loss: A randomized controlled trial. *FASEB Journal* 27 (9): 3837-3847.

Portal, S., Zadik, Z., Rabinowitz, J., et al. 2011. The effect of HMB supplementation on body composition, fitness, hormonal and inflammatory mediators in elite adolescent volleyball players: A prospective randomized, double-blind, placebo-controlled study. *European Journal of Applied Physiology* 111 (9): 2261-2269.

Racette, Susan B. 2003. Creatine supplementation and athletic performance. *Journal of Orthopaedic & Sports Physical Therapy* 33 (10): 615-621.

Reissig, Chad A. 2009. Caffeinated energy drinks—a growing problem. *Drug and Alcohol Dependence* 99 (1-3): 1-10.

Rivera-Brown, A., Gutierrez, R., Gutierrez, J.C., et al. 1999. Drink composition, voluntary drinking, and fluid balance in exercising, trained, heat-acclimatized boys. *Journal of Applied Physiology* 86 (1): 78-84.

Rogol, A.D., Roemmich, J.N., and Clark, P.A. 2002. Growth at puberty. *Journal of Adolescent Health* 31 (6 Suppl.): 192-200.

Rosenbloom, Christine, et al. 2012. *Sports nutrition: A practical manual for professionals,* 5th ed. Academy of Nutrition and Dietetics. Chicago, Illinois.

Rowland, T. 2011. Fluid replacement requirements for child athletes. *Sports Medicine* 41 (4): 279-288.

Salinero, J.J., et al. 2014. The use of energy drinks in sport: Perceived ergogenic and side effects in male and female athlete. *British Journal of Nutrition* 112 (9): 1494-1502.

Sarubin Fragakis, Allison, and Thomson, Cynthia A. 2006. Food sources of creatine. In *The health professional's guide to popular dietary supplements,* 3rd ed., 142-143. Academy of Nutrition and Dietetics. Chicago, Illinois.

Saugy, M., et al. 2006. Human growth hormone doping in sport. *British Journal of Sports Medicine* 40 (Suppl. 1): i35-i39.

Schafer, Michael. 2006. Ephedra use in a select group of adolescent athletes. *Journal of Sports Science & Medicine* 5 (3): 407-414.

Sciberras, Joseph, et al. 2015. The effect of turmeric (curcumin) supplementation on cytokine and inflammatory marker responses following 2 hours of endurance cycling. *Journal of the International Society of Sports Nutrition* 12 (1): 5.

Scott, A.T. 2015. Improvement of 2000-m rowing performance with caffeinated carbohydrate-gel ingestion. *International Journal of Sports Physiology and Performance* 10 (4): 464-468.

Seifert, S.M., et al. 2013. An analysis of energy-drink toxicity in the National Poison Data System. *Clinical Toxicology* 51 (7): 566-574.

Serrano, E., et al. 2010. Antioxidant defence and inflammatory response in professional road cyclists during a 4-day competition. *Journal of Sports Science* 28 (10): 1047-1056.

Shei, R.J. 2014. Omega-3 polyunsaturated fatty acids in the optimization of physical performance. *Military Medicine* 179 (11 Suppl.): 144-156.

Sinclair, Lisa, and Hinton, Pamela Sue. 2005. Prevalence of iron deficiency with and without anemia in recreationally active men and women. *Journal of the American Dietetic Association* 105 (6): 975-978.

Skinner, Tina, et al. 2010. Dose response of caffeine on 2000-m rowing performance. *Medicine & Science in Sports & Exercise* 42 (3): 571-576.

Smith, J., and Dahm, D.L. 2000. Creatine use among a select population of high school athletes. *Mayo Clinic Proceedings* 75 (12): 1257-1263.

Smith, J.W., Holmes, M.E., and McAllister, M.J. 2015. Nutritional considerations for performance in young athletes. *Journal of Sports Medicine* 2015: 734649.

Smith, Rachel, et al. 2104. A review of creatine supplementation in age-related diseases: More than a supplement for athletes. *F1000Research* 15 (3): 222.

Smith T, Lynch M.E. and Johnson James. Herbal Dietary Supplements Sales in US Increases 6.8% in 2004. HerbalGram, American Botanical Council; Austin, Texas. 2015; Issue: 107; Page 52-59.

Snijders, T., Res, P.T., and Smeets, J.S. 2015. Protein ingestion before sleep increases muscle mass and strength gains during prolonged resistance-type exercise training in healthy young men. *Journal of Nutrition* 145 (6): 1178-1184.

Song, Q.H. 2015. Glutamine supplementation and immune function during heavy load training. *International Journal of Clinical Pharmacology* 5 (5): 372-376.

Spaccarotella, K.J., and Andzel, W.D. 2011. The effects of low fat chocolate milk on postexercise recovery in collegiate athletes. *Journal of Strength and Conditioning Research* 25 (12): 3456-3460.

Stang, J., and Story, M. 2005. Adolescent growth and development. In *Guidelines for adolescent nutrition services,* edited by J. Stang and M. Story, 1-8.

Stevenson, Emma, et al. 2009. The effect of a carbohydrate-caffeine sports drink on stimulated golf performance. Applied Physiology, Nutrition, and Metabolism 34 (4): 681-688.

Supplement Safety Now. www.supplementsafetynow.com.

Supplement Watch. www.supplementwatch.com.

Tamminen, K.A., Holt, N.L., and Crocker P.R.E. 2012. Adolescent athletes: Psychological challenges and clinical concerns. *Current Opinion in Psychiatry* 25: 293-300.

Tanner, J.M. 1962. *Growth at adolescence.* Oxford: Blackwell Scientific Publications.

Tartibian, B. 2010. The effects of omega-3 supplementation on pulmonary function of young wrestlers during intensive training. *Journal of Science and Medicine in Sport* 13 (2): 281-286.

Taylor Hooton Foundation. (n.d.). Steroid abuse among kids. http://taylorhooton.org/wp-content/themes/taylorhooton/images/Fact-Sheet.pdf.

The International Olympic Committee (IOC). www.olympic.org/ioc.

Thomas, K., Morris, P., and Stevenson, E. 2009. Improved endurance capacity following chocolate milk consumption compared with 2 commercially available sport drinks. *Applied Physiology, Nutrition, and Metabolism* 34 (1): 78-82.

Tokmakidis, S.P., and Karamanolis, I.A. 2008. Effect of carbohydrate ingestion 15 min before exercise on endurance running capacity. *Applied Physiology, Nutrition, and Metabolism* 33 (3): 441-449.

Too, B.W., Cicai, S., Hockett, K.R., et al. 2012. Natural versus commercial carbohydrate supplementation and endurance running performance. *Journal of the International Society of Sports Nutrition* 9 (1): 27.

Torun, Benjamin. 2005. Energy requirements of children and adolescents. *Public Health Nutrition* 8 (7A): 968-993.

United Nations University, World Health Organization, and Food and Agriculture Organization of the United Nations. 2004, October 17-24. Energy requirements of children and adolescents. In *Human energy requirements,* 20-34. Rome: Food and Agriculture Organization of the United Nations.

U.S. Anti-Doping Agency (USADA), TrueSport. www.usada.org/truesport.

U.S. Centers for Disease Control and Prevention. (n.d.). 2 to 20 years: Boys body mass index-for-age percentile. www.cdc.gov/growthcharts/data/set1clinical/cj41l023.pdf.

U.S. Centers for Disease Control and Prevention. 2 to 20 years: Girls body mass index-for-age percentile. www.cdc.gov/growthcharts/data/set1clinical/cj41l024.pdf.

U.S. Department of Agriculture. (n.d.). ChooseMyPlate.gov. www.choosemyplate.gov

U.S. Department of Agriculture. (n.d.). USDA food composition database. https://ndb.nal.usda.gov.

U.S. Department of Agriculture, Food and Nutrition Services. 2012. Nutrition standards in the National School Lunch and School Breakfast programs. *Federal Register 77* (17). www.gpo.gov/fdsys/pkg/FR-2012-01-26/pdf/2012-1010.pdf

U.S. Department of Health and Human Services, and U.S. Department of Agriculture. 2015. *2015-2020 Dietary Guidelines for Americans,* 8th ed. http://health.gov/dietaryguidelines/2015/guidelines.

U.S. Food and Drug Administration. Center for Food Safety and Applied Nutrition (CFSAN) Adverse Event Reporting System (CAERS). https://www.nationalacademies.org/hmd/~/media/Files/Activity%20Files /Nutrition/PotentialEffectsofCaffeine/CAERS_Adverse-Events-Report.pdf.

U.S. Food and Drug Administration. (n.d.). 1994 Dietary Supplement Health and Education Act (DSHEA). https://ods.od.nih.gov/About/DSHEA_Wording.aspx.

U.S. Food and Drug Administration. 2014. FDA investigation summary: Acute hepatitis illnesses linked to certain OxyElite Pro products. www.fda.gov/Food/RecallsOutbreaksEmergencies/Outbreaks/ucm370849.htm.

U.S. Pharmacopeial (USP). www.usp.org.

Valimaki, V., Alfthan, H., Lehmuskallio, E., et al. 2005. Risk factors for clinical stress factors in male military recruits: A prospective cohort study. *Bone* 37 (2): 267-273.

Weiss, Alison, Xu, Fang, Storfer-Isser, Amy, et al. 2010. The association of sleep duration with adolescents' fat and carbohydrate consumption. *Sleep* 33 (9): 1201-1209.

Whitehead MT, Martin TD, Scheett TP, et al. Running economy and maximal oxygen consumption after 4 weeks of oral Echinacea supplementation. *J Strength Cond Res* 2012;26:1928-33

Wilk, B., Timmons, B., and Bar-Or, O. 2010. Voluntary fluid intake hydration status and aerobic performance. *Applied Physiology, Nutrition, and Metabolism* 35 (6): 834-841.

Willis, K.S., Peterson, N.J., and Larson-Meyer, D.E. 2008. Should we be concerned about the vitamin D status of athletes? *International Journal of Sport Nutrition and Exercise Metabolism* 18 (2): 204-224.

Wilson, Jacob, Fitschen, Peter, Campbell, Bill, et al. 2013. International Society of Sports Nutrition position stand: Beta-hydroxy-beta-methylbutyrate (HMB). *Journal of the International Society of Sports Nutrition* 10: 6.

Woolf, K., St Thomas, M.M., Hahn, N., et al. 2009. Iron status in highly active and sedentary young women. *International Journal of Sport Nutrition and Exercise Metabolism* 19 (5): 519-535.

World Anti-Doping Agency. www.USADA.org.

Index

Note: Page references followed by an italicized *f* or *t* indicate information contained in figures or tables, respectively.

About the Author

Heather Mangieri, MS, RDN, CSSD, LDN, is an award-winning food and nutrition expert, registered dietitian, and board-certified specialist in sport dietetics. She is the founder of Nutrition CheckUp, a nutrition consulting practice with expertise in sport nutrition, weight management, and disordered eating. She consults with a variety of clients, including casual exercisers, competitive athletes, and families looking to eat well while navigating busy schedules. She specializes in helping active adolescents eat well for proper growth, development, and sport performance.

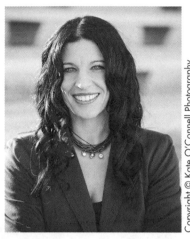

Copyright © Kate O'Connell Photography

Since 2010 Mangieri has been a national media spokesperson for the Academy of Nutrition and Dietetics. She has built a reputation for delivering evidence-based messages in sport nutrition, adolescent sport nutrition, weight management, ergogenic aids, dietary supplements, fad diets, and lifestyle modification. Mangieri frequently writes about sport nutrition in the professional publications of the National Collegiate Athletic Association and the Academy of Nutrition and Dietetics as well as in *Stack* magazine and *Food and Nutrition* magazine. She has been quoted in hundreds of national publications, including *Fitness, ESPNW, ESPN Kids, Runner's World, Women's Running, Women's Health, Men's Fitness, Men's Health, New York Times, Chicago Tribune, Los Angeles Times,* and *USA Today.* In addition to national recognition, she has a strong local following, appearing frequently on KDKA Pittsburgh's show *Night Talk.*

Mangieri speaks regularly to athletes, consumers, and professionals about sport nutrition, dietary supplements, weight management, and disordered eating. In June 2014 she spoke on disordered eating in athletes at the first Eating Disorders in Sport conference and spoke on the same topic at the 2015 annual meeting of the Collegiate & Professional Sports Dietitians Association.

In 2008 Mangieri was recognized as Pennsylvania's Young Dietitian of the Year. In 2012 she received the Keystone award in recognition of her leadership in demonstrating outstanding professional standards to serve and advance the aim of Pennsylvania dietitians. She serves on the executive committee of Sports, Cardiovascular, and Wellness Nutrition (SCAN), a dietary practice group of the Academy of Nutrition and Dietetics.

Mangieri studied human nutrition with an emphasis on research at Pennsylvania State University, earning a BS degree in 1996. She earned her master's degree from the University of Pittsburgh in wellness and human performance in 2007. Before entering private practice, she was an instructor at the University of Pittsburgh in the department of sports medicine and nutrition and a part-time faculty member in the department of exercise science at Chatham University, teaching nutrition and exercise classes to undergraduate students.

Mangieri lives in the Pittsburgh metropolitan area.

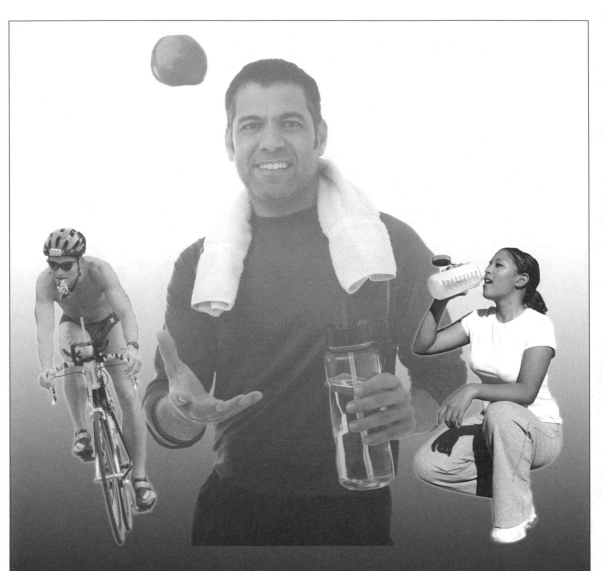

You'll find other outstanding sports nutrition resources at

www.HumanKinetics.com/nutritionandhealthyeating

In the U.S. call 1-800-747-4457

Australia 08 8372 0999 • Canada 1-800-465-7301
Europe +44 (0) 113 255 5665 • New Zealand 0800 222 062

HUMAN KINETICS
The Premier Publisher for Sports & Fitness
P.O. Box 5076 • Champaign, IL 61825-5076 USA

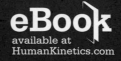

eBook
available at
HumanKinetics.com